Virtual Clinical Excursions

for

Cooper and Gosnell:
Foundations and Adult Health Nursing
8th Edition

Virtual Clinical Excursions

for

Cooper and Gosnell:
Foundations and Adult Health Nursing
8th Edition

prepared by

Jennifer Morris, RN, BSN
Assistant Professor of Vocational Nursing
South Plains College
Levelland, Texas

software developed by

Wolfsong Informatics, LLC
Tucson, Arizona

ELSEVIER

ELSEVIER

3251 Riverport Lane
Maryland Heights, Missouri 63043

VIRTUAL CLINICAL EXCURSIONS FOR
COOPER AND GOSNELL:
FOUNDATIONS AND ADULT HEALTH NURSING
8TH EDITION

ISBN: 978-0-323-52444-5

Notice

Knowledge and best practice in this field are constantly changing. As new research and experience broaden our understanding, changes in research methods, professional practices, or medical treatment may become necessary.

Practitioners and researchers must always rely on their own experience and knowledge in evaluating and using any information, methods, compounds, or experiments described herein. In using such information or methods they should be mindful of their own safety and the safety of others, including parties for whom they have a professional responsibility.

With respect to any drug or pharmaceutical products identified, readers are advised to check the most current information provided (i) on procedures featured or (ii) by the manufacturer of each product to be administered, to verify the recommended dose or formula, the method and duration of administration, and contraindications. It is the responsibility of practitioners, relying on their own experience and knowledge of their patients, to make diagnoses, to determine dosages and the best treatment for each individual patient, and to take all appropriate safety precautions.

To the fullest extent of the law, neither the Publisher nor the authors, contributors, or editors, assume any liability for any injury and/or damage to persons or property as a matter of products liability, negligence or otherwise, or from any use or operation of any methods, products, instructions, or ideas contained in the material herein.

ISBN: 978-0-323-52444-5

Printed in the United States of America

Last digit is the print number: 9 8 7 6 5 4 3 2

Workbook
prepared by

Jennifer Morris, RN, BSN
Assistant Professor of Vocational Nursing
South Plains College
Levelland, Texas

Textbook

Kim Cooper, RN, MSN
Associate Professor and Dean, School of Nursing
Ivy Tech Community College
Terre Haute, Indiana

President, Indiana Board of Nursing

Kelly Gosnell, RN, MSN
Associate Professor and Department Chair
School of Nursing
Ivy Tech Community College
Terre Haute, Indiana

Table of Contents
Virtual Clinical Excursions Workbook

Table of Contents
Cooper and Gosnell:
Foundations and Adult Health Nursing, 8th Edition

GETTING SET UP WITH VCE ONLINE ─────────────

The product you have purchased is part of Evolve. Please read the following information thoroughly to get started.

■ HOW TO ACCESS YOUR VCE RESOURCES ON EVOLVE

There are a few ways to access your VCE Resources on Evolve:

1. If your instructor has enrolled you in your VCE Evolve Resources, you will receive an email with your registration details, depending on the learning management system (LMS) your instructor is using.

2. If your instructor has asked you to self-enroll in your VCE Evolve Resources on the Evolve LMS, he or she will provide you with your Course ID (for example, 1479_jdoe73_0001). You will then need to enter your Course ID at https://evolve.elsevier.com/cs/store?role=student.

3. If your school uses a different LMS (e.g., Blackboard, Moodle, or Brightspace), please check with your instructor or institution's LMS administrator on how to enroll in the course.

■ HOW TO ACCESS THE ONLINE VIRTUAL HOSPITAL

The online virtual hospital is available through the Evolve VCE Resources. There is no software to download or install: the online virtual hospital runs within your Internet browser, using a pop-up window.

■ TECHNICAL REQUIREMENTS

- Broadband connection (DSL or cable)
- 1024 x 768 screen resolution
- Mozilla Firefox, Internet Explorer 11, Google Chrome, Edge, or Safari
  Note: Pop-up blocking software/settings must be disabled.
- Adobe Acrobat Reader
- Additional technical requirements available at http://evolvesupport.elsevier.com

■ HOW TO ACCESS THE WORKBOOK

There are two ways to access the workbook portion of *Virtual Clinical Excursions:*

1. Print workbook
2. An electronic version of the workbook, available within the VCE Evolve Resources

■ TECHNICAL SUPPORT

Technical support for *Virtual Clinical Excursions* is available by visiting the Technical Support Center at http://evolvesupport.elsevier.com or by calling 1-800-222-9570 inside the United States and Canada.

Trademarks: Windows® and Macintosh® are registered trademarks.

A QUICK TOUR

Welcome to *Virtual Clinical Excursions*, a virtual hospital setting in which you can work with multiple complex patient simulations and also learn to access and evaluate the information resources that are essential for high-quality patient care. The virtual hospital, Pacific View Regional Hospital, has realistic architecture and access to patient rooms, a Nurses' Station, and a Medication Room.

■ BEFORE YOU START

Make sure you have your textbook nearby when you use *Virtual Clinical Excursions*. You will want to consult topic areas in your textbook frequently while working with the virtual hospital and workbook.

■ HOW TO SIGN IN

- Enter your name on the Student Nurse identification badge.
- Next, specify the floor on which you will work by clicking the down arrow next to **Select Floor**. For this quick tour, choose **Medical-Surgical**.
- Now choose one of the four periods of care in which to work. In Periods of Care 1 through 3, you can actively engage in patient assessment, entry of data in the electronic patient record (EPR), and medication administration. Period of Care 4 presents the day in review. Highlight and click the appropriate period of care. (For this quick tour, choose **Period of Care 1: 0730-0815**.)
- This takes you to the Patient List screen (see the **How to Select a Patient** section below). Only the patients on the Medical-Surgical Floor are available. Note that the virtual time is provided in the box at the lower left corner of the screen (0730, since we chose Period of Care 1).

Note: If you choose to work during Period of Care 4: 1900-2000, the Patient List screen is skipped since you are not able to visit patients or administer medications during the shift. Instead, you are taken directly to the Nurses' Station, where the records of all the patients on the floor are available for your review.

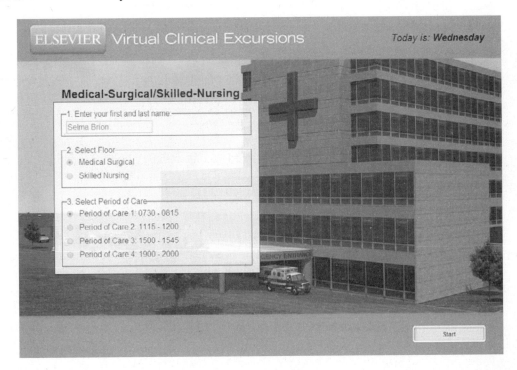

■ PATIENT LIST

MEDICAL-SURGICAL UNIT

Harry George (Room 401)
Osteomyelitis—A 54-year-old Caucasian male admitted from a homeless shelter with an infected leg. He has complications of type 2 diabetes mellitus, alcohol abuse, nicotine addiction, poor pain control, and complex psychosocial issues.

Jacquline Catanazaro (Room 402)
Asthma—A 45-year-old Caucasian female admitted with an acute asthma exacerbation and suspected pneumonia. She has complications of chronic schizophrenia, noncompliance with medication therapy, obesity, and herniated disc.

Piya Jordan (Room 403)
Bowel obstruction—A 68-year-old Asian female admitted with a colon mass and suspected adenocarcinoma. She undergoes a right hemicolectomy. This patient's complications include atrial fibrillation, hypokalemia, and symptoms of meperidine toxicity.

Clarence Hughes (Room 404)
Degenerative joint disease—A 73-year-old African-American male admitted for a left total knee replacement. His preparations for discharge are complicated by the development of a pulmonary embolus and the need for ongoing intravenous therapy.

Pablo Rodriguez (Room 405)
Metastatic lung carcinoma—A 71-year-old Hispanic male admitted with symptoms of dehydration and malnutrition. He has chronic pain secondary to multiple subcutaneous skin nodules and psychosocial concerns related to family issues with his approaching death.

Patricia Newman (Room 406)
Pneumonia—A 61-year-old Caucasian female admitted with worsening pulmonary function and an acute respiratory infection. Her chronic emphysema is complicated by heavy smoking, hypertension, and malnutrition. She needs access to community resources such as a smoking cessation program and meal assistance.

SKILLED NURSING UNIT

William Jefferson (Room 501)
Alzheimer's disease—A 75-year-old African-American male admitted for stabilization of type 2 diabetes and hypertension following a recent acute care admission for a urinary tract infection and sepsis. His complications include episodes of acute delirium and a history of osteoarthritis.

Delores Gallegos (Room 502)
Congestive heart failure—An 82-year-old Hispanic female admitted to the Skilled Nursing Unit for congestive heart failure. During her stay it is determined that she has dermatitis, as well as emerging pneumonia.

Kathryn Doyle (Room 503)
Rehabilitation post left hip replacement—A 79-year-old Caucasian female admitted following a complicated recovery from an ORIF. She is experiencing symptoms of malnutrition and depression due to unstable family dynamics, placing her at risk for elder abuse.

Carlos Reyes (Room 504)

Rehabilitation status post myocardial infarction—An 81-year-old Hispanic male admitted for evaluation of the need for long-term care following an acute care hospital stay. Recent cognitive changes and a diagnosis of anxiety disorder contribute to stressful family dynamics and care-giver strain.

Goro Oishi (Room 505)

Hospice care—A 66-year-old Asian male admitted following an acute care admission for an intracerebral hemorrhage and resulting coma. Family-staff interactions provide opportunities to explore death and dying issues related to conflict about advanced life support and cultural and religious differences.

■ HOW TO SELECT A PATIENT

- You can choose one or more patients to work with from the Patient List by checking the box to the left of the patient name(s). For this quick tour, select Piya Jordan and Pablo Rodriguez. (In order to receive a scorecard for a patient, the patient must be selected before proceeding to the Nurses' Station.)
- Click on **Get Report** to the right of the medical records number (MRN) to view a summary of the patient's care during the 12-hour period before your arrival on the unit.
- After reviewing the report, click on **Go to Nurses' Station** in the right lower corner to begin your care. (*Note:* If you have been assigned to care for multiple patients, you can click on **Return to Patient List** to select and review the report for each additional patient before going to the Nurses' Station.)

Note: Even though the Patient List is initially skipped when you sign in to work for Period of Care 4, you can still access this screen if you wish to review the shift report for any of the patients. To do so, simply click on **Patient List** near the top left corner of the Nurses' Station (or click on the clipboard to the left of the Kardex). Then click on **Get Report** for the patient(s) whose care you are reviewing. This may be done during any period of care.

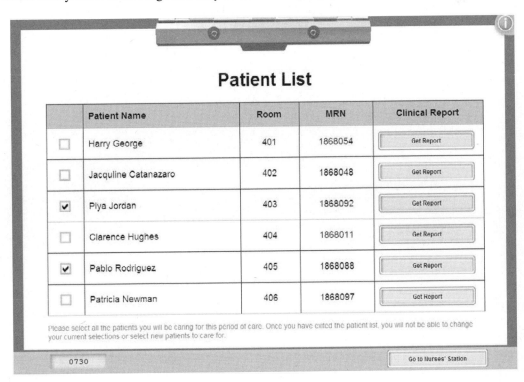

Patient List

	Patient Name	Room	MRN	Clinical Report
☐	Harry George	401	1868054	Get Report
☐	Jacquline Catanazaro	402	1868048	Get Report
☑	Piya Jordan	403	1868092	Get Report
☐	Clarence Hughes	404	1868011	Get Report
☑	Pablo Rodriguez	405	1868088	Get Report
☐	Patricia Newman	406	1868097	Get Report

Please select all the patients you will be caring for this period of care. Once you have exited the patient list, you will not be able to change your current selections or select new patients to care for.

0730

Go to Nurses' Station

■ HOW TO FIND A PATIENT'S RECORDS

NURSES' STATION

Within the Nurses' Station, you will see:

1. A clipboard that contains the patient list for that floor.
2. A chart rack with patient charts labeled by room number, a notebook labeled Kardex, and a notebook labeled MAR (Medication Administration Record).
3. A desktop computer with access to the Electronic Patient Record (EPR).
4. A tool bar across the top of the screen that can also be used to access the Patient List, EPR, Chart, MAR, and Kardex. This tool bar is also accessible from each patient's room.
5. A Drug Guide containing information about the medications you are able to administer to your patients.
6. A Laboratory Guide containing normal value ranges for all laboratory tests you may come across in the virtual patient hospital.
7. A tool bar across the bottom of the screen that can be used to access the Floor Map, patient rooms, Medication Room, and Drug Guide.

As you run your cursor over an item, it will be highlighted. To select, simply click on the item. As you use these resources, you will always be able to return to the Nurses' Station by clicking on the **Return to Nurses' Station** bar located in the right lower corner of your screen.

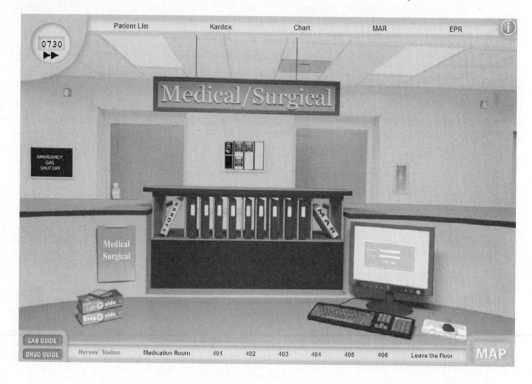

MEDICATION ADMINISTRATION RECORD (MAR)

The MAR icon located on the tool bar at the top of your screen accesses current 24-hour medications for each patient. Click on the icon and the MAR will open. (*Note:* You can also access the MAR by clicking on the MAR notebook on the far right side of the book rack in the center of the screen.) Within the MAR, tabs on the right side of the screen allow you to select patients by room number. Be careful to make sure you select the correct tab number for *your* patient rather than simply reading the first record that appears after the MAR opens. Each MAR sheet lists the following:

- Medications
- Route and dosage of each medication
- Times of administration of each medication

Note: The MAR changes each day. Expired MARs are stored in the patients' charts.

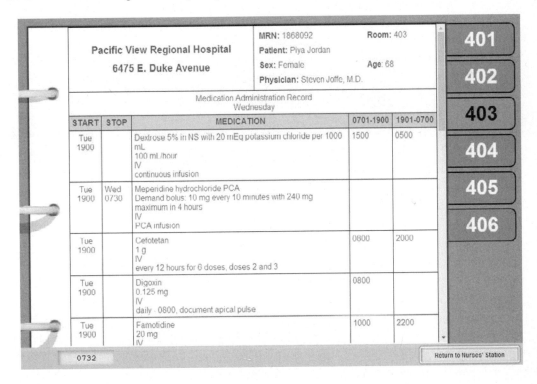

CHARTS

To access patient charts, either click on the **Chart** icon at the top of your screen or anywhere within the chart rack in the center of the Nurses' Station screen. When the close-up view appears, the individual charts are labeled by room number. To open a chart, click on the room number of the patient whose chart you wish to review. The patient's name and allergies will appear on the left side of the screen, along with a list of tabs on the right side of the screen, allowing you to view the following data:

- Allergies
- Physician's Orders
- Physician's Notes
- Nurse's Notes
- Laboratory Reports
- Diagnostic Reports
- Surgical Reports
- Consultations

- Patient Education
- History and Physical
- Nursing Admission
- Expired MARs
- Consents
- Mental Health
- Admissions
- Emergency Department

Information appears in real time. The entries are in reverse chronologic order, so use the down arrow at the right side of each chart page to scroll down to view previous entries. Flip from tab to tab to view multiple data fields or click on **Return to Nurses' Station** in the lower right corner of the screen to exit the chart.

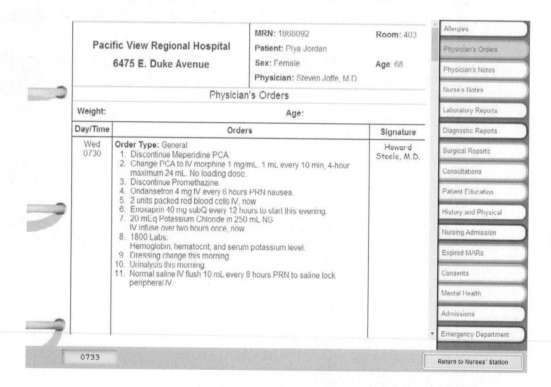

ELECTRONIC PATIENT RECORD (EPR)

The EPR can be accessed from the computer in the Nurses' Station or from the EPR icon located in the tool bar at the top of your screen. To access a patient's EPR:
- Click on either the computer screen or the **EPR** icon.
- Your username and password are automatically filled in.
- Click on **Login** to enter the EPR.
- *Note:* Like the MAR, the EPR is arranged numerically. Thus when you enter, you are initially shown the records of the patient in the lowest room number on the floor. To view the correct data for *your* patient, remember to select the correct room number, using the drop-down menu for the Patient field at the top left corner of the screen.

The EPR used in Pacific View Regional Hospital represents a composite of commercial versions being used in hospitals. You can access the EPR:
- to review existing data for a patient (by room number).
- to enter data you collect while working with a patient.

The EPR is updated daily, so no matter what day or part of a shift you are working, there will be a current EPR with the patient's data from the past days of the current hospital stay. This type of simulated EPR allows you to examine how data for different attributes have changed over time, as well as to examine data for all of a patient's attributes at a particular time. The EPR is fully functional (as it is in a real-life hospital). You can enter such data as blood pressure, breath sounds, and certain treatments. The EPR will not, however, allow you to enter data for a previous time period. Use the arrows at the bottom of the screen to move forward and backward in time.

Name: Piya Jordan	Wed 0630	Wed 0700	Wed 0715	Code Meanings
PAIN: LOCATION		OS		
PAIN: RATING		5		
PAIN: CHARACTERISTICS		C		
PAIN: VOCAL CUES		VC3		
PAIN: FACIAL CUES		FC1		
PAIN: BODILY CUES				
PAIN: SYSTEM CUES				
PAIN: FUNCTIONAL EFFECTS				
PAIN: PREDISPOSING FACTORS				
PAIN: RELIEVING FACTORS				
PCA		P		
TEMPERATURE (F)		99.6		
TEMPERATURE (C)				
MODE OF MEASUREMENT		Ty		
SYSTOLIC PRESSURE		110		
DIASTOLIC PRESSURE		70		
BP MODE OF MEASUREMENT		NIBP		
HEART RATE		104		
RESPIRATORY RATE		18		
SpO2 (%)		95		
BLOOD GLUCOSE				
WEIGHT				
HEIGHT				

Patient: 403 · Category: Vital Signs · 0735 · Return to Nurses' Station

At the top of the EPR screen, you can choose patients by their room numbers. In addition, you have access to 17 different categories of patient data. To change patients or data categories, click the down arrow to the right of the room number or category.

The categories of patient data in the EPR are as follows:

- Vital Signs
- Respiratory
- Cardiovascular
- Neurologic
- Gastrointestinal
- Excretory
- Musculoskeletal
- Integumentary
- Reproductive
- Psychosocial
- Wounds and Drains
- Activity
- Hygiene and Comfort
- Safety
- Nutrition
- IV
- Intake and Output

Remember, each hospital selects its own codes. The codes used in the EPR at Pacific View Regional Hospital may be different from ones you have seen in your clinical rotations. Take some time to acquaint yourself with the codes. Within the Vital Signs category, click on any item in the left column (e.g., Pain: Characteristics). In the far-right column, you will see a list of code meanings for the possible findings and/or descriptors for that assessment area.

You will use the codes to record the data you collect as you work with patients. Click on the box in the last time column to the right of any item and wait for the code meanings applicable to that entry to appear. Select the appropriate code to describe your assessment findings and type it in the box. (*Note:* If no cursor appears within the box, click on the box again until the blue shading disappears and the blinking cursor appears.) Once the data are typed in this box, they are entered into the patient's record for this period of care only.

To leave the EPR, click on **Exit EPR** in the bottom right corner of the screen.

■ VISITING A PATIENT

From the Nurses' Station, click on the room number of the patient you wish to visit (in the tool bar at the bottom of your screen). Once you are inside the room, you will see a still photo of your patient in the top left corner. To verify that this is the correct patient, click on the **Check Armband** icon to the right of the photo. The patient's identification data will appear. If you click on **Check Allergies** (the next icon to the right), a list of the patient's allergies (if any) will replace the photo.

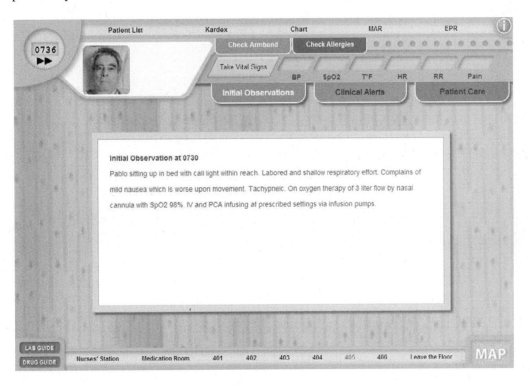

Also located in the patient's room are multiple icons you can use to assess the patient or the patient's medications. A virtual clock is provided in the upper left corner of the room to monitor your progress in real time. (*Note:* The fast-forward icon within the virtual clock will advance the time by 2-minute intervals when clicked.)

- The tool bar across the top of the screen allows you to check the **Patient List**, access the **EPR** to check or enter data, and view the patient's **Chart**, **MAR**, or **Kardex**.

- The **Take Vital Signs** icon allows you to measure the patient's up-to-the-minute blood pressure, oxygen saturation, temperature, heart rate, respiratory rate, and pain level.

- Each time you enter a patient's room, you are given an Initial Observation report to review (in the text box under the patient's photo). These notes are provided to give you a "look" at the patient as if you had just stepped into the room. You can also click on the **Initial Observations** icon to return to this box from other views within the patient's room. To the right of this icon is **Clinical Alerts**, a resource that allows you to make decisions about priority medication interventions based on emerging data collected in real time. Check this screen throughout your period of care to avoid missing critical information related to recently ordered or STAT medications.

- Clicking on **Patient Care** opens up three specific learning environments within the patient room: **Physical Assessment**, **Nurse-Client Interactions**, and **Medication Administration**.

- To perform a **Physical Assessment**, choose a body area (such as **Head & Neck**) from the column of yellow buttons. This activates a list of system subcategories for that body area (e.g., see **Sensory**, **Neurologic**, etc. in the green boxes). After you select the system you wish to evaluate, a brief description of the assessment findings will appear in a box to the right. A still photo provides a "snapshot" of how an assessment of this area might be done or what the finding might look like. For every body area, you can also click on **Equipment** on the right side of the screen.

- To the right of the Physical Assessment icon is **Nurse-Client Interactions**. Clicking on this icon will reveal the times and titles of any videos available for viewing. (*Note:* If the video you wish to see is not listed, this means you have not yet reached the correct virtual time to view that video. Check the virtual clock; you may return to access the video once its designated time has occurred—as long as you do so within the same period of care. Or you can click on the fast-forward icon within the virtual clock to advance the time by 2-minute intervals. You will then need to click again on **Patient Care** and **Nurse-Client Interactions** to refresh the screen.) To view a listed video, click on the white arrow to the right of the video title. Use the control buttons below the video to start, stop, pause, rewind, or fast-forward the action or to mute the sound.

- **Medication Administration** is the pathway that allows you to review and administer medications to a patient after you have prepared them in the Medication Room. This process is also addressed further in the *How to Prepare Medications* section below and in *Medications* in the **Detailed Tour**. For additional hands-on practice, see *Reducing Medication Errors* below the **Quick Tour** and the **Detailed Tour** in your resources.

■ HOW TO QUIT, CHANGE PATIENTS, OR CHANGE PERIODS OF CARE

How to Quit: From most screens, you may click the **Leave the Floor** icon on the bottom tool bar to the right of the patient room numbers. (*Note:* From some screens, you will first need to click an **Exit** button or **Return to Nurses' Station** before clicking **Leave the Floor**.) When the Floor Menu appears, click **Exit** to leave the program.

How to Change Patients or Periods of Care: To change patients, simply click on the new patient's room number. (You cannot receive a scorecard for a new patient, however, unless you have already selected that patient on the Patient List screen.) To change to a new period of care or to restart the virtual clock, click on **Leave the Floor** and then on **Restart the Program**.

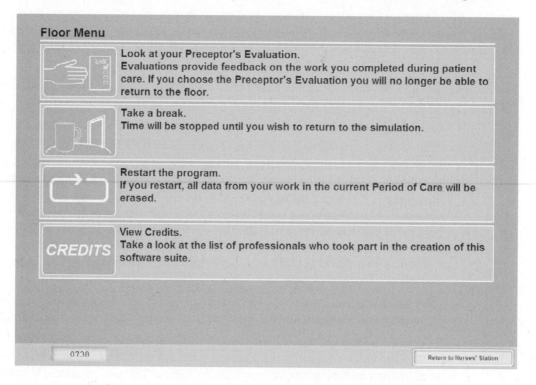

■ HOW TO PREPARE MEDICATIONS

From the Nurses' Station or the patient's room, you can access the Medication Room by clicking on the icon in the tool bar at the bottom of your screen to the left of the patient room numbers.

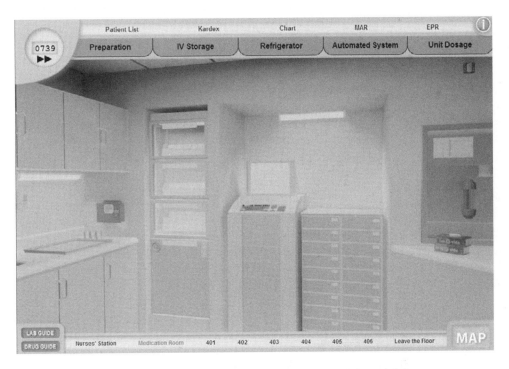

In the Medication Room you have access to the following (from left to right):

- A preparation area is located on the counter under the cabinets. To begin the medication preparation process, click on the tray on the counter or click on the **Preparation** icon at the top of the screen. The next screen leads you through a specific sequence (called the Preparation Wizard) to prepare medications one at a time for administration to a patient. However, no medication has been selected at this time. We will do this while working with a patient in **A Detailed Tour**. To exit this screen, click on **View Medication Room**.

- To the right of the cabinets (and above the refrigerator), IV storage bins are provided. Click on the bins themselves or on the **IV Storage** icon at the top of the screen. The bins are labeled **Microinfusion**, **Small Volume**, and **Large Volume**. Click on an individual bin to see a list of its contents. If you needed to prepare an IV medication at this time, you could click on the medication and its label would appear to the right under the patient's name. (*Note:* You can **Open** and **Close** any medication label by clicking the appropriate icon.) Next, you would click **Put Medication on Tray**. If you ever change your mind or decide that you have put the incorrect medication on the tray, you can reverse your actions by highlighting the medication on the tray and then clicking **Put Medication in Bin**. Click **Close Bin** in the right bottom corner to exit. **View Medication Room** brings you back to a full view of the entire room.

- A refrigerator is located under the IV storage bins to hold any medications that must be stored below room temperature. Click on the refrigerator door or on the **Refrigerator** icon at the top of the screen. Then click on the close-up view of the door to access the medications. When you are finished, click **Close Door** and then **View Medication Room**.

- To prepare controlled substances, click the **Automated System** icon at the top of the screen or click the computer monitor located to the right of the IV storage bins. A login screen will appear; your name and password are automatically filled in. Click **Login**. Select the patient for whom you wish to access medications; then select the correct medication drawer to open (they are stored alphabetically). Click **Open Drawer**, highlight the proper medication, and choose **Put Medication on Tray**. When you are finished, click **Close Drawer** and then **View Medication Room**.

- Next to the Automated System is a set of drawers identified by patient room number. To access these, click on the drawers or on the **Unit Dosage** icon at the top of the screen. This provides a close-up view of the drawers. To open a drawer, click on the room number of the patient you are working with. Next, click on the medication you would like to prepare for the patient, and a label will appear, listing the medication strength, units, and dosage per unit. To exit, click **Close Drawer**; then click **View Medication Room**.

At any time, you can learn about a medication you wish to prepare for a patient by clicking on the **Drug** icon in the bottom left corner of the medication room screen or by clicking the **Drug Guide** book on the counter to the right of the unit dosage drawers. The **Drug Guide** provides information about the medications commonly included in nursing drug handbooks. Nutritional supplements and maintenance intravenous fluid preparations are not included. Highlight a medication in the alphabetical list; relevant information about the drug will appear in the screen below. To exit, click **Return to Medication Room**.

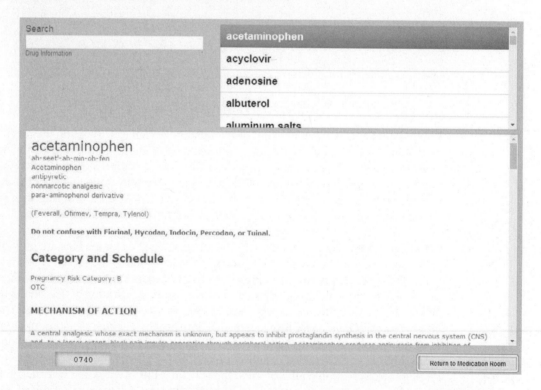

To access the MAR from the Medication Room and to review the medications ordered for a patient, click on the **MAR** icon located in the tool bar at the top of your screen and then click on the correct tab for your patient's room number. You may also click the **Review MAR** icon in the tool bar at the bottom of your screen from inside each medication storage area.

After you have chosen and prepared medications, go to the patient's room to administer them by clicking on the room number in the bottom tool bar. Inside the patient's room, click **Patient Care** and then **Medication Administration** and follow the proper administration sequence.

■ PRECEPTOR'S EVALUATIONS

When you have finished a session, click on **Leave the Floor** to go to the Floor Menu. At this point, you can click on the top icon (**Look at Your Preceptor's Evaluation**) to receive a score-card that provides feedback on the work you completed during patient care.

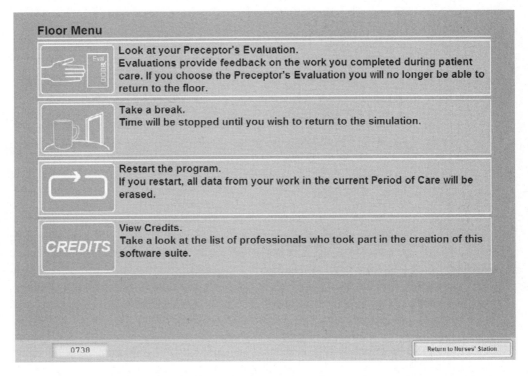

Evaluations are available for each patient you selected when you signed in for the current period of care. Click on the **Medication Scorecard** icon to see an example.

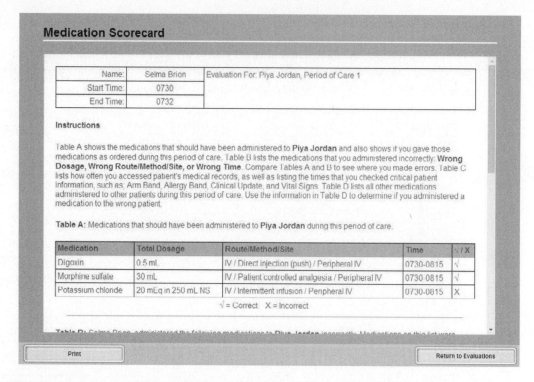

The scorecard compares the medications you administered to a patient during a period of care with what should have been administered. Table A lists the correct medications. Table B lists any medications that were administered incorrectly.

Remember, not every medication listed on the MAR should necessarily be given. For example, a patient might have an allergy to a drug that was ordered, or a medication might have been improperly transcribed to the MAR. Predetermined medication "errors" embedded within the program challenge you to exercise critical thinking skills and professional judgment when deciding to administer a medication, just as you would in a real hospital. Use all your available resources, such as the patient's chart and the MAR, to make your decision.

Table C lists the resources that were available to assist you in medication administration. It also documents whether and when you accessed these resources. For example, did you check the patient armband or perform a check of vital signs? If so, when?

You can click **Print** to get a copy of this report if needed. When you have finished reviewing the scorecard, click **Return to Evaluations** and then **Return to Menu**.

■ FLOOR MAP

To get a general sense of your location within the hospital, you can click on the **Map** icon found in the lower right corner of most of the screens in the *Virtual Clinical Excursions—Skilled Nursing* or *Medical-Surgical* program. (*Note:* If you are following this quick tour step by step, you will need to **Restart the Program** from the Floor Menu, sign in again, and go to the Nurses' Station to access the map.) When you click the **Map** icon, a floor map appears, showing the layout of the floor you are currently on, as well as a directory of the patients and services on that floor. As you move your cursor over the directory list, the location of each room is highlighted on the map (and vice versa). The floor map can be accessed from the Nurses' Station, Medication Room, and each patient's room.

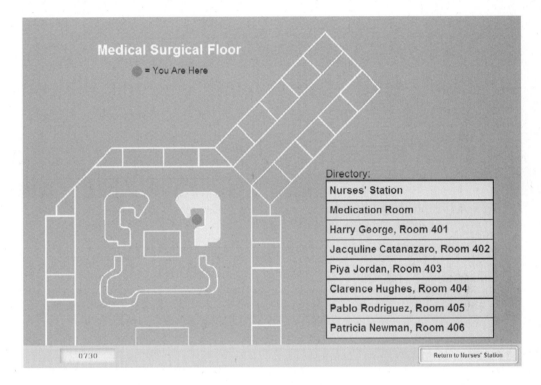

A DETAILED TOUR

If you wish to more thoroughly understand the capabilities of *Virtual Clinical Excursions*, take a detailed tour by completing the following section. During this tour, we will work with a specific patient to introduce you to all the different components and learning opportunities available within the software.

■ WORKING WITH A PATIENT

Sign in and select the Medical-Surgical Floor for Period of Care 1 (0730-0815). From the Patient List, select Piya Jordan and Pablo Rodriguez; however, do not go to the Nurses' Station yet.

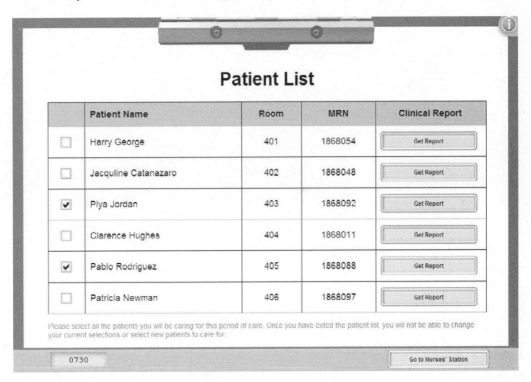

■ REPORT

In hospitals, when one shift ends and another begins, the outgoing nurse who attended a patient will give a verbal and sometimes a written summary of that patient's condition to the incoming nurse who will assume care for the patient. This summary is called a report and is an important source of data to provide an overview of a patient. Your first task is to get the clinical report on Piya Jordan. To do this, click **Get Report** in the far right column in this patient's row. From a brief review of this summary, identify the problems and areas of concern that you will need to address for this patient.

When you have finished noting any areas of concern, click **Go to Nurses' Station**.

■ CHARTS

You can access Piya Jordan's chart from the Nurses' Station or from the patient's room (403). From the Nurses' Station, click on the chart rack or on the **Chart** icon in the tool bar at the top of your screen. Next, click on the chart labeled **403** to open the medical record for Piya Jordan. Click on the **Emergency Department** tab to view a record of why this patient was admitted.

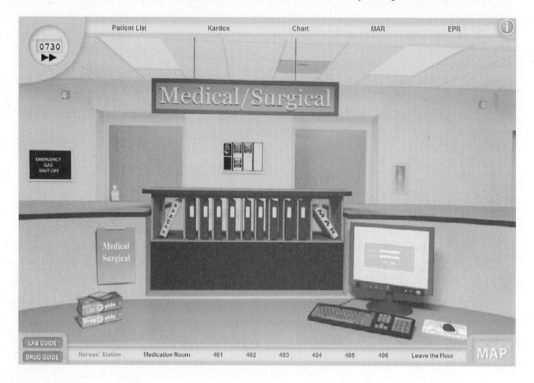

How many days has Piya Jordan been in the hospital?

What tests were done upon her arrival in the Emergency Department and why?

What was her reason for admission?

You should also click on **Diagnostic Reports** to learn what additional tests or procedures were performed and when. Finally, review the **Nursing Admission** and **History and Physical** to learn about the health history of this patient. When you are done reviewing the chart, click **Return to Nurses' Station**.

■ MEDICATIONS

Open the Medication Administration Record (MAR) by clicking on the **MAR** icon in the tool bar at the top of your screen. *Remember:* The MAR automatically opens to the first occupied room number on the floor—which is not necessarily your patient's room number! Since you need to access Piya Jordan's MAR, click on tab **403** (her room number). Always make sure you are giving the *Right Drug to the Right Patient!*

Examine the list of medications ordered for Piya Jordan. In the table below, list the medications that need to be given during this period of care (0730-0815). For each medication, note the dosage, route, and time to be given.

Time	Medication	Dosage	Route

Click on **Return to Nurses' Station**. Next, click on **403** on the bottom tool bar and then verify that you are indeed in Piya Jordan's room. Select **Clinical Alerts** (the icon to the right of Initial Observations) to check for any emerging data that might affect your medication administration priorities. Next, go to the patient's chart (click on the **Chart** icon; then click on **403**). When the chart opens, select the **Physician's Orders** tab.

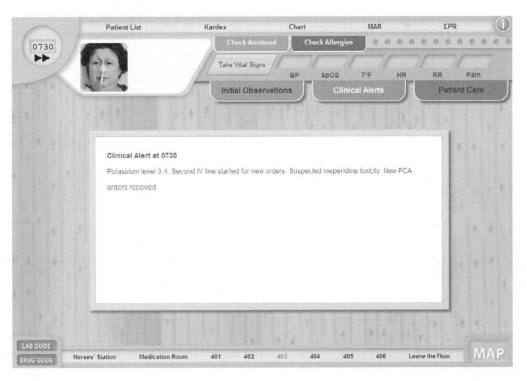

Review the orders. Have any new medications been ordered? Return to the MAR (click **Return to Room 403**; then click **MAR**). Verify that any new medications have been correctly transcribed to the MAR. Mistakes are sometimes made in the transcription process in the hospital setting, and it is sound practice to double-check any new order.

Are there any patient assessments you will need to perform before administering these medications? If so, return to Room 403 and click on **Patient Care** and then **Physical Assessment** to complete those assessments before proceeding.

Now click on the **Medication Room** icon in the tool bar at the bottom of your screen to locate and prepare the medications for Piya Jordan.

In the Medication Room, you must access the medications for Piya Jordan from the specific dispensing system in which each medication is stored. Locate each medication that needs to be given in this time period and click on **Put Medication on Tray** as appropriate. (*Hint:* Look in **Unit Dosage** drawer first.) When you are finished, click on **Close Drawer** and then on **View Medication Room**. Now click on the medication tray on the counter on the left side of the medication room screen to begin preparing the medications you have selected. (*Remember:* You can also click **Preparation** in the tool bar at the top of the screen.)

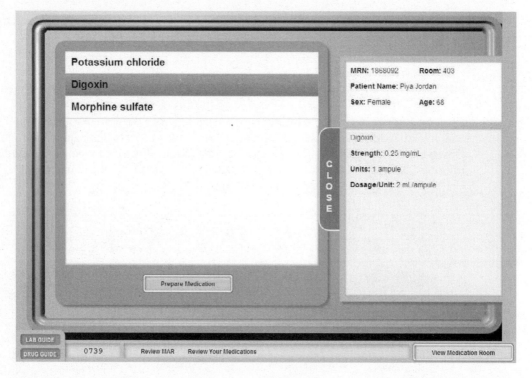

In the preparation area, you should see a list of the medications you put on the tray in the previous steps. Click on the first medication and then click **Prepare**. Follow the onscreen instructions of the Preparation Wizard, providing any data requested. As an example, let's follow the preparation process for digoxin, one of the medications due to be administered to Piya Jordan during this period of care. To begin, click to select **Digoxin**; then click **Prepare**. Now work through the Preparation Wizard sequence as detailed below:

> Amount of medication in the ampule: 2 mL.
> Enter the amount of medication you will draw up into a syringe: **0.5** mL.
> Click **Next**.
> Select the patient you wish to set aside the medication for: **Room 403, Piya Jordan**.
> Click **Finish**.
> Click **Return to Medication Room**.

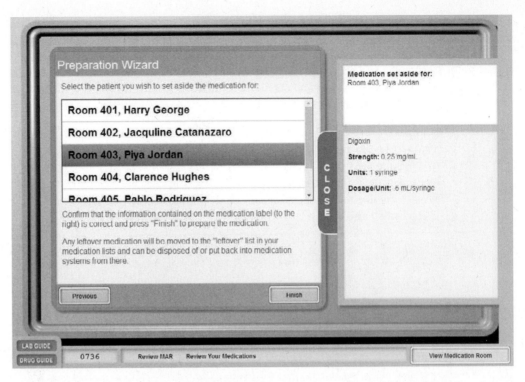

Follow this same basic process for the other medications due to be administered to Piya Jordan during this period of care. (*Hint:* Look in **IV Storage** and **Automated System**.)

PREPARATION WIZARD EXCEPTIONS

- Some medications in *Virtual Clinical Excursions* are preprepared by the pharmacy (e.g., IV antibiotics) and taken to the patient room as a whole. This is common practice in most hospitals.
- Blood products are not administered by students through the *Virtual Clinical Excursions* simulations since blood administration follows specific protocols not covered in this program.
- The *Virtual Clinical Excursions* simulations do not allow for mixing more than one type of medication, such as regular and Lente insulins, in the same syringe. In the clinical setting, when multiple types of insulin are ordered for a patient, the regular insulin is drawn up first, followed by the longer-acting insulin. Insulin is always administered in a special unit-marked syringe.

Now return to Room 403 (click on **403** on the bottom tool bar) to administer Piya Jordan's medications.

At any time during the medication administration process, you can perform a further review of systems, take vital signs, check information contained within the chart, or verify patient identity and allergies. Inside Piya Jordan's room, click **Take Vital Signs**. (*Note:* These findings change over time to reflect the temporal changes you would find in a patient similar to Piya Jordan.)

When you have gathered all the data you need, click on **Patient Care** and then select **Medication Administration**. Any medications you prepared in the previous steps should be listed on the left side of your screen. Let's continue the administration process with the digoxin ordered for Piya Jordan. Click to highlight **Digoxin** in the list of medications. Next, click on the down arrow to the right of **Select** and choose **Administer** from the drop-down menu. This will activate the Administration Wizard. Complete the Wizard sequence as follows:

- Route: **IV**
- Method: **Direct Injection**
- Site: **Peripheral IV**
- Click **Administer to Patient** arrow.
- Would you like to document this administration in the MAR? **Yes**
- Click **Finish** arrow.

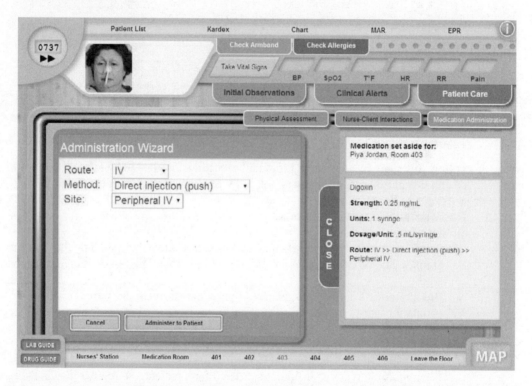

Your selections are recorded by a tracking system and evaluated on a Medication Scorecard stored under Preceptor's Evaluations. This scorecard can be viewed, printed, and given to your instructor. To access the Preceptor's Evaluations, click on **Leave the Floor**. When the Floor Menu appears, select **Look at Your Preceptor's Evaluation**. Then click on **Medication Scorecard** inside the box with Piya Jordan's name (see example on the following page).

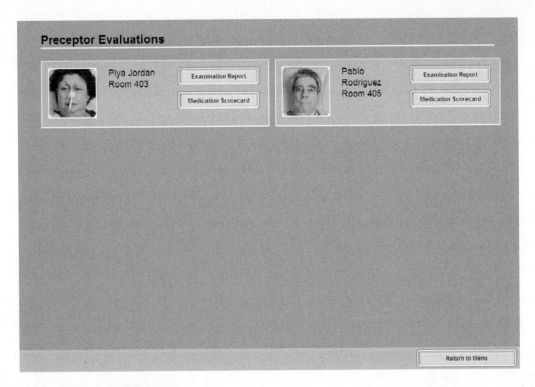

■ MEDICATION SCORECARD

- First, review Table A. Was digoxin given correctly? Did you give the other medications as ordered?
- Table B shows you which (if any) medications you gave incorrectly.
- Table C addresses the resources used for Piya Jordan. Did you access the patient's chart, MAR, EPR, or Kardex as needed to make safe medication administration decisions?
- Did you check the patient's armband to verify her identity? Did you check whether your patient had any known allergies to medications? Were vital signs taken?

When you have finished reviewing the scorecard, click **Return to Evaluations** and then **Return to Menu**.

■ **VITAL SIGNS**

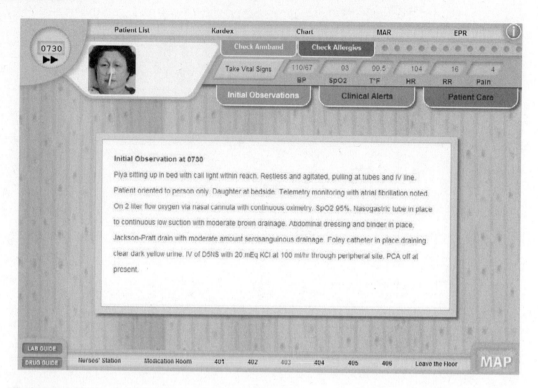

Vital signs, often considered the traditional "signs of life," include body temperature, heart rate, respiratory rate, blood pressure, oxygen saturation of the blood, and pain level.

Inside Piya Jordan's room, click **Take Vital Signs**. (*Note:* If you are following this detailed tour step by step, you will need to **Restart the Program** from the Floor Menu, sign in again for Period of Care 1, and navigate to Room 403.) Collect vital signs for this patient and record them below. Note the time at which you collected each of these data. (*Remember:* You can take vital signs at any time. The data change over time to reflect the temporal changes you would find in a patient similar to Piya Jordan.)

Vital Signs	Findings/Time
Blood pressure	
O$_2$ saturation	
Temperature	
Heart rate	
Respiratory rate	
Pain rating	

After you are done, click on the **EPR** icon located in the tool bar at the top of the screen. Your username and password are automatically provided. Click on **Login** to enter the EPR. To access Piya Jordan's records, click on the down arrow next to Patient and choose her room number, **403**. Select **Vital Signs** as the category. Next, in the empty time column on the far right, record the vital signs data you just collected in Piya Jordan's room. If you need help with this process, refer to the Electronic Patient Record (EPR) section of the Quick Tour. Now compare these findings with the data you collected earlier for this patient's vital signs. Use these earlier findings to establish a baseline for each of the vital signs.

    a.   Are any of the data you collected significantly different from the baseline for a particular vital sign?

        Circle One: Yes   No

    b.   If "Yes," which data are different?

■ PHYSICAL ASSESSMENT

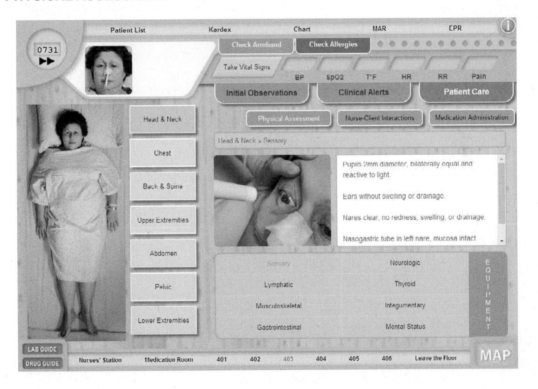

After you have finished examining the EPR for vital signs, click **Exit EPR** to return to Room 403. Click **Patient Care** and then **Physical Assessment**. Think about the information you received in the report at the beginning of this shift, as well as what you may have learned about this patient from the chart. Based on this, what area(s) of examination should you pay most attention to at this time? Is there any equipment you should be monitoring? Conduct a physical assessment of the body areas and systems that you consider priorities for Piya Jordan. For example, select **Head & Neck**; then click on and assess **Sensory** and **Lymphatic**. Complete any other assessment(s) you think are necessary at this time. In the following table, record the data you collected during this examination.

Area of Examination	Findings
Head & Neck Sensory	
Head & Neck Lymphatic	

After you have finished collecting these data, return to the EPR. Compare the data that were already in the record with those you just collected.

    a. Are any of the data you collected significantly different from the baselines for this patient?

        Circle One: Yes   No

    b. If "Yes," which data are different?

■ NURSE-CLIENT INTERACTIONS

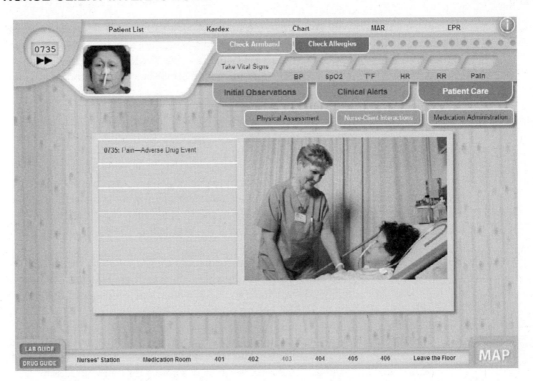

Click on **Patient Care** from inside Piya Jordan's room (403). Now click on **Nurse-Client Interactions** to access a short video titled **Pain—Adverse Drug Event**, which is available for viewing at or after 0735 (based on the virtual clock in the upper left corner of your screen; see *Note* below). To begin the video, click on the arrow next to its title. You will observe a nurse communicating with Piya Jordan and her daughter. There are many variations of nursing practice, some exemplifying "best" practice and some not. Note whether the nurse in this interaction displays professional behavior and compassionate care. Are her words congruent with what is going on with the patient? Does this interaction "feel right" to you? If not, how would you handle this situation differently? Explain.

Note: If the video you wish to view is not listed, this means you have not yet reached the correct virtual time to view that video. Check the virtual clock; you may return to access the video once its designated time has occurred—as long as you do so within the same period of care. Or you can click on the fast-forward icon within the virtual clock to advance the time by 2-minute intervals. You will then need to click again on **Patient Care** and **Nurse-Client Interactions** to refresh the screen.

At least one Nurse-Client Interactions video is available during each period of care. Viewing these videos can help you learn more about what is occurring with a patient at a certain time and also prompt you to discern between nurse communications that are ideal and those that need improvement. Compassionate care and the ability to communicate clearly are essential components of delivering quality nursing care, and it is during your clinical time that you will begin to refine these skills.

■ COLLECTING AND EVALUATING DATA

Each of the activities you perform in the Patient Care environment generates a significant amount of assessment data. Remember that after you collect data, you can record your findings in the EPR. You can also review the EPR, patient's chart, videos, and MAR at any time. You will get plenty of practice collecting and then evaluating data in context of the patient's course.

Now, here's an important question for you:

> Did the previous sequence of exercises provide the most efficient way to assess Piya Jordan?

For example, you went to the patient's room to get vital signs, then back to the EPR to enter data and compare your findings with extant data. Next, you went back to the patient's room to do a physical examination, then again back to the EPR to enter and review data. If this back-and-forth process of data collection and recording seemed inefficient, remember the following:

- Plan all of your nursing activities to maximize efficiency, while at the same time optimizing the quality of patient care. (Think about what data you might need before performing certain tasks. For example, do you need to check a heart rate before administering a cardiac medication or check an IV site before starting an infusion?)

- You collect a tremendous amount of data when you work with a patient. Very few people can accurately remember all these data for more than a few minutes. Develop efficient assessment skills, and record data as soon as possible after collecting them.

- Assessment data are only the starting point for the nursing process.

Make a clear distinction between these first exercises and how you actually provide nursing care. These initial exercises were designed to involve you actively in the use of different software components. This workbook focuses on sensible practices for implementing the nursing process in ways that ensure the highest-quality care of patients.

Most important, remember that a human being changes through time, and that these changes include both the physical and psychosocial facets of a person as a living organism. Think about this for a moment. Some patients may change physically in a very short time (a patient with emerging myocardial infarction) or more slowly (a patient with a chronic illness). Patients' overall physical and psychosocial conditions may improve or deteriorate. They may have effective coping skills and familial support, or they may feel alone and full of despair. In fact, each individual is a complex mix of physical and psychosocial elements, and at least some of these elements usually change through time.

Thus it is crucial that you *DO NOT* think of the nursing process as a simple one-time, five-step procedure consisting of assessment, nursing diagnosis, planning, implementation, and evaluation. Rather, the nursing process should be utilized as a creative and systematic approach to delivering nursing care. Furthermore, because all living organisms are constantly changing, we must apply the nursing process over and over. Each time we follow the nursing process for an individual patient, we refine our understanding of that patient's physical and psychosocial conditions based on collection and analysis of many different types of data. *Virtual Clinical Excursions* will help you develop both the creativity and the systematic approach needed to become a nurse who is equipped to deliver the highest-quality care to all patients.

REDUCING MEDICATION ERRORS

Earlier in the detailed tour, you learned the basic steps of medication preparation and administration. The following simulations will allow you to practice those skills further—with an increased emphasis on reducing medication errors by using the Medication Scorecard to evaluate your work.

Sign in to work at Pacific View Regional Hospital for Period of Care 1. (*Note:* If you are already working with another patient or during another period of care, click on **Leave the Floor** and then **Restart the Program**; then sign in.)

From the Patient List, select Clarence Hughes. Then click on **Go to Nurses' Station**. Complete the following steps to prepare and administer medications to Clarence Hughes.

- Click on **Medication Room** on the tool bar at the bottom of your screen.
- Click on **MAR** and then on tab **404** to determine medications that have been ordered for Clarence Hughes. (*Note:* You may click on **Review MAR** at any time to verify the correct medication order. Always remember to check the patient name on the MAR to make sure you have the correct patient's record. You must click on the correct room number tab within the MAR.) Click on **Return to Medication Room** after reviewing the correct MAR.
- Click on **Unit Dosage** (or on the Unit Dosage cabinet); from the close-up view, click on drawer **404**.
- Select the medications you would like to administer. After each selection, click **Put Medication on Tray**. When you are finished selecting medications, click **Close Drawer** and then **View Medication Room**.
- Click on **Automated System** (or on the Automated System unit itself). Click **Login**.
- On the next screen, specify the correct patient and drawer location.
- Select the medication you would like to administer and click on **Put Medication on Tray**. Repeat this process if you wish to administer other medications from the Automated System.
- When you are finished, click **Close Drawer** and **View Medication Room**.
- From the Medication Room, click on **Preparation** (or on the preparation tray).
- From the list of medications on your tray, highlight the correct medication to administer and click **Prepare**.
- This activates the Preparation Wizard. Supply any requested information; then click **Next**.
- Now select the correct patient to receive this medication and click **Finish**.
- Repeat the previous three steps until all medications that you want to administer are prepared.
- You can click on **Review Your Medications** and then on **Return to Medication Room** when ready. Once you are back in the Medication Room, go directly to Clarence Hughes' room by clicking on **404** at bottom of screen.
- Inside the patient's room, administer the medication, utilizing the six rights of medication administration. After you have collected the appropriate assessment data and are ready for administration, click **Patient Care** and then **Medication Administration**. Verify that the correct patient and medication(s) appear in the left-hand window. Highlight the first medication you wish to administer; then click the down arrow next to Select. From the drop-down menu, select **Administer** and complete the Administration Wizard by providing any information requested. When the Wizard stops asking for information, click **Administer to Patient**. Specify **Yes** when asked whether this administration should be recorded in the MAR. Finally, click **Finish**.

■ **SELF-EVALUATION**

Now let's see how you did during your medication administration!

- Click on **Leave the Floor** at the bottom of your screen. From the Floor Menu, select **Look at Your Preceptor's Evaluation**. Then click **Medication Scorecard**.

The following exercises will help you identify medication errors, investigate possible reasons for these errors, and reduce or prevent medication errors in the future.

1. Start by examining Table A. These are the medications you should have given to Clarence Hughes during this period of care. If each of the medications in Table A has a ✓ by it, then you made no errors. Congratulations!

If any medication has an X by it, then you made one or more medication errors.

Compare Tables A and B to determine which of the following types of errors you made: Wrong Dose, Wrong Route/Method/Site, or Wrong Time. Follow these steps:
   a. Find medications in Table A that were given incorrectly.
   b. Now see if those same medications are in Table B, which shows what you actually administered to Clarence Hughes.
   c. Comparing Tables A and B, match the Strength, Dose, Route/Method/Site, and Time for each medication you administered incorrectly.
   d. Then, using the form below, list the medications given incorrectly and mark the errors you made for each medication.

Medication	Strength	Dosage	Route	Method	Site	Time
	❏	❏	❏	❏	❏	❏
	❏	❏	❏	❏	❏	❏
	❏	❏	❏	❏	❏	❏
	❏	❏	❏	❏	❏	❏

2. To help you reduce future medication errors, consider the following list of possible reasons for errors.

   - Did not check drug against MAR for correct medication, correct dose, correct patient, correct route, correct time, correct documentation.
   - Did not check drug dose against MAR three times.
   - Did not open the unit dose package in the patient's room.
   - Did not correctly identify the patient using two identifiers.
   - Did not administer the drug on time.
   - Did not verify patient allergies.
   - Did not check the patient's current condition or vital sign parameters.
   - Did not consider why the patient would be receiving this drug.
   - Did not question why the drug was in the patient's drawer.
   - Did not check the physician's order and/or check with the pharmacist when there was a question about the drug or dose.
   - Did not verify that no adverse effects had occurred from a previous dose.

Based on the list of possibilities you just reviewed, determine how you made each error and record the reason in the form below:

Medication	Reason for Error

3. Look again at Table B. Are there medications listed that are not in Table A? If so, you gave a medication to Clarence Hughes that he should not have received. Complete the following exercises to help you understand how such an error might have been made.

   a. Perhaps you gave a medication that was on Clarence Hughes' MAR for this period of care, without recognizing that a change had occurred in the patient's condition, which should have caused you to reconsider. Review patient records as necessary and complete the following form:

Medication	Possible Reasons Not to Give This Medication

   b. Another possibility is that you gave Clarence Hughes a medication that should have been given at a different time. Check his MAR and complete the form below to determine whether you made a Wrong Time error:

Medication	Given to Clarence Hughes at What Time	Should Have Been Given at What Time

c. Maybe you gave another patient's medication to Clarence Hughes. In this case, you made a Wrong Patient error. Check the MARs of other patients and use the form below to determine whether you made this type of error:

Medication	Given to Clarence Hughes	Should Have Been Given to

4. The Medication Scorecard provides some other interesting sources of information. For example, if there is a medication selected for Clarence Hughes but it was not given to him, there will be an X by that medication in Table A, but it will not appear in Table B. In that case, you might have given this medication to some other patient, which is another type of Wrong Patient error. To investigate further, look at Table D, which lists the medications you gave to other patients. See whether you can find any medications ordered for Clarence Hughes that were given to another patient by mistake. However, before you make any decisions, be sure to cross-check the MAR for other patients because the same medication may have been ordered for multiple patients. Use the following form to record your findings:

Medication	Should Have Been Given to Clarence Hughes	Given by Mistake to

5. Now take some time to review the medication exercises you just completed. Use the form below to create an overall analysis of what you have learned. Once again, record each of the medication errors you made, including the type of each error. Then, for each error you made, indicate specifically what you would do differently to prevent this type of error from occurring again.

Medication	Type of Error	Error Prevention Tactic

Submit this form to your instructor if required as a graded assignment, or simply use these exercises to improve your understanding of medication errors and how to reduce them.

Name: _____   Date: _____

LESSON 1

An Overview of Communication Barriers

Reading Assignment: Communication (Chapter 4)

Patient: William Jefferson, Room 501

Objectives:

1. Identify the factors that may hinder nurse-patient interactions.
2. List the communication tools necessary to successfully interact with cognitively impaired patients.
3. Discuss three styles of communication.
4. Understand the rationale for nursing interventions used to successfully communicate with cognitively impaired patients.

Exercise 1

Writing Activity

30 minutes

1. List some obstacles that may affect interactions between nurses and older adults.

2. List several techniques that the nurse should use when interacting with patients who are cognitively impaired. (*Hint:* See Box 4-4 in your textbook.)

3. What are some guidelines for a nurse to follow in order to effectively communicate with an older adult?

4. Discuss methods that may be used to communicate with hearing-impaired patients. (*Hint:* See Box 4-5 in your textbook.)

5. The two types of communication are _____ and _____.

6. List the elements of nonverbal communication. (*Hint:* See Table 4-1 in your textbook.)

7. A therapeutic nurse-patient interaction is needed to promote quality care. Which elements foster a therapeutic nurse-client relationship? Select all that apply.

_____ Hugging

_____ Sincerity

_____ Empathy

_____ Trustworthiness

_____ Sympathy

_____ Demonstrating parental behaviors toward the patient

_____ Caring attitude

8. _____ refers to a communication technique that incorporates the feelings and needs of the patient.

9. _____ communication occurs when an individual interacts with another in an overpowering and forceful manner.

10. Which nursing behaviors demonstrate cultural awareness? Select all that apply.

    _____ Maintain eye contact during the interaction.

    _____ Use touch, as appropriate for the interaction, after the patient's comfort level has been assessed.

    _____ Call the patient by his or her first name to promote feelings of familiarity and closeness.

    _____ Assess contextual speech patterns of the group.

    _____ Identify the patient's personal spatial and distancing preferences.

11. When using touch to communicate with a patient, what must the nurse take into consideration?

12. What should a nurse understand regarding acceptance for a patient's beliefs and/or decisions?

13. When using humor during a patient interaction, which of the following guidelines must the nurse remember?
    a. The nurse must be aware of when humor is appropriate and when it is inappropriate.
    b. Humor should not be used during periods of emotional grief.
    c. The nurse should be the party leading the interaction and determining when the use of humor is appropriate.
    d. Humor should not be used during periods in which the patient is experiencing pain.

Exercise 2

Virtual Hospital Activity

15 minutes

- Sign in to work at Pacific View Regional Hospital for Period of Care 1. (*Note:* If you are already in the virtual hospital from a previous exercise, click on **Leave the Floor** and then **Restart the Program** to get to the sign-in window.)
- From the Patient List, select William Jefferson (Room 501).
- Click **Get Report** and read the Clinical Report.
- Click **Go to Nurses' Station**.
- Click **501** at the bottom of the screen to go to the patient's room.
- Read the **Initial Observations**.

1. What psychosocial issues could create barriers to the nurse's interaction with William Jefferson? How might these issues affect the interaction?

2. What physiologic and environmental issues being experienced by William Jefferson may affect the nurse-patient interaction?

3. When the nurse is communicating with William Jefferson, which interventions will help to establish a positive rapport? Select all that apply.

_____ Assisting the patient to the dining room to promote feelings of socialization

_____ Facing the patient during the interaction

_____ Avoiding analgesic administration to reduce drowsiness during the interaction

_____ Providing adequate lighting during the exchange

_____ Using touch as culturally appropriate

4. When caring for William Jefferson, the nurse knows that which variable will have the most influence on communication?
   a. His age and race
   b. His culture and social position
   c. The scheduled agenda for the day
   d. The race of the care provider
   e. Disorientation and confusion

5. William Jefferson is confused and getting dressed to take his dog for a walk. What action by the nurse is most appropriate?
   a. Assist him to dress with the hope that this task will distract him.
   b. Explain that his dog is not at the hospital with him.
   c. Ignore the confusion and respond with factual information.
   d. Show him a photo of his dog.

Exercise 3

Virtual Hospital Activity

15 minutes

- Sign in to work at Pacific View Regional Hospital for Period of Care 2. (*Note:* If you are already in the virtual hospital from a previous exercise, click on **Leave the Floor** and then **Restart the Program** to get to the sign-in window.)
- From the Patient List, select William Jefferson (Room 501).
- Click on **Get Report** and read the Clinical Report.

1. What cognitive changes have taken place in William Jefferson during the last shift?

2. What behavioral manifestations are occurring as a result of these changes?

- Click **Go to Nurses' Station**.
- Click **501** at the bottom of the screen to enter the patient's room.
- Review the **Initial Observations**.
- Click **Patient Care** and then **Nurse-Client Interactions**.
- Select and view the video titled **1115: Team Communication**. (*Note:* Check the virtual clock to see whether enough time has elapsed. You can use the fast-forward feature to advance the time by 2-minute intervals if the video is not yet available. Then click again on **Patient Care** and **Nurse-Client Interactions** to refresh the screen.)

3. What three planned nursing interventions that were discussed in the team conference will be implemented by the nurse?

4. Give a rationale for each of the above planned interventions.

- Select and view the video titled **1120: The Agitated Patient**. (*Note:* Check the virtual clock to see whether enough time has elapsed. You can use the fast-forward feature to advance the time by 2-minute intervals if the video is not yet available. Then click again on **Patient Care** and **Nurse-Client Interactions** to refresh the screen.)

5. In the video, what verbal communication technique does the nurse use in her interaction with William Jefferson?

6. What were the nonverbal cues used during the nurse's interaction with the patient?

7. What did the nurse do to reinforce William Jefferson's mental orientation?

Exercise 4

Virtual Hospital Activity

10 minutes

- Sign in to work at Pacific View Regional Hospital for Period of Care 3. (*Note:* If you are already in the virtual hospital from a previous exercise, click on **Leave the Floor** and then **Restart the Program** to get to the sign-in window.)
- From the Patient List, select William Jefferson (Room 501).
- Click **Get Report** and read the Clinical Report.
- Click **Go to Nurses' Station**.
- Click **501** at the bottom of the screen to go to the patient's room.
- Read the **Initial Observations**.

- Click **Patient Care** and then click **Nurse-Client Interactions**.
- Select and view the video titled **1525: Living with Alzheimer's**. (*Note:* Check the virtual clock to see whether enough time has elapsed. You can use the fast-forward feature to advance the time by 2-minute intervals if the video is not yet available. Then click again on **Patient Care** and **Nurse-Client Interactions** to refresh the screen.)

1. List four nonverbal cues that will affect an exchange of information between two individuals.

2. Review the exchange between William Jefferson and the student nurse. Is the posture exhibited best described as open or closed? Provide a rationale for your choice.

3. The student nurse in the interaction has demonstrated therapeutic/assertive communication skills. Identify the specific tools used by the nurse in the video. Select all that apply.

   _____ Appears composed

   _____ Maintains eye contact

   _____ Uses touch

   _____ Uses silence

   _____ Uses active listening

4. During the interaction between the student nurse, the patient, and the patient's wife, which communication technique is used most by the student?
   a. Open-ended questioning
   b. Clarifying
   c. Paraphrasing
   d. Restating

5. When interacting with William Jefferson, eye contact can impact the success of the interaction. The nurse must be mindful of the nonverbal messages made by eye contact. If William Jefferson maintains constant eye contact, what should the nurse consider a likely interpretation?
   a. William Jefferson is experiencing a degree of increasing anxiety during the encounter.
   b. The steady eye contact signals potential aggression.
   c. The encounter may be causing him to feel threatened.
   d. No inferences can be made from the level of eye contact.

The Nursing Process

Reading Assignment: Nursing Process and Critical Thinking (Chapter 5)

Patient: William Jefferson, Room 501

Objectives:

1. Identify sources of data when developing a plan of care.
2. Discuss the differences between nursing and medical diagnoses.
3. Apply the principles of the nursing process.
4. Prioritize the patient concerns by level of importance.

Exercise 1

Writing Activity

15 minutes

1. Explain the differences between subjective and objective data.

2. In addition to the patient, who and/or what are some other sources of data?

3. What is the purpose of a nursing diagnosis? What are the four components of a nursing diagnosis?

4. How do medical and nursing diagnoses differ?

5. Match each aspect of the nursing process with its appropriate description.

Nursing Process Aspect	Description
_____ Assess	a. Set goals of care and desired outcomes
_____ Plan and identify outcomes	b. Identify the patient's problems
_____ Implement	c. Gather information about the patient's condition
_____ Evaluate	d. Determine whether goals have been met and outcomes have been achieved
_____ Diagnose	e. Perform the nursing actions identified during planning

6. For each assessment finding, identify the type of data.

Assessment Finding	Type of Data
_____ Grimaces with pain when touched	a. Objective data
_____ Reports feeling fatigue	b. Subjective data
_____ Temperature 100.7	
_____ Alert and oriented during assessment	
_____ Hemoglobin 12.2 mg/dL	

Exercise 2

Virtual Hospital Activity

45 minutes

- Sign in to work at Pacific View Regional Hospital for Period of Care 3. (*Note:* If you are already in the virtual program from a previous exercise, click on **Leave the Floor** and then **Restart the Program** to get to the sign-in window.)
- From the Patient List, select William Jefferson (Room 501).
- Click **Get Report** and read the Clinical Report.
- Click **Go to Nurses' Station**.
- Click **Chart** and then click **501** to see William Jefferson's chart.
- Click the **Nursing Admission** tab and read the report.

1. Who appears to be the primary provider of information in the nursing admission assessment of William Jefferson?

2. Identify the primary concerns reported by the patient.

3. Which health concerns have been identified as medical diagnoses for William Jefferson? Select all that apply.

_____ Alzheimer's disease

_____ Stress incontinence

_____ Urinary tract infection

_____ Hypertension

_____ Potential for anxiety

_____ Osteoarthritis

_____ Type 2 diabetes

_____ Diabetes insipidus

_____ Resolving sepsis

- Click the **History and Physical** tab and review the report.

4. Based on information you have reviewed in the Nursing Admission and the History and Physical, identify several areas of concern for William Jefferson.

5. For three of the above areas of concern, develop a possible nursing diagnosis.

6. _____ statements are based on the desired patient-driven expectations.

7. Patient-driven outcomes are referred to as _____.

8. The system used to prioritize the needs of a patient, with physiologic needs before those

   focusing on love and belonging, is known as _____.

9. Listed are the identified areas of concern for William Jefferson. Rank them in order of importance.

Area of Concern	Order of Importance
_____ Potential for reinfection	a. First
_____ Management and stabilization of hypertension	b. Second
_____ Management and stabilization of diabetes mellitus	c. Third
_____ Management of confusion	d. Fourth

10. Develop a patient outcome relating to William Jefferson's potential for injury.

11. Develop a patient outcome relating to William Jefferson's diabetes mellitus.

12. How do nursing interventions and physician-prescribed interventions differ?

- Still in the patient's chart, click the **Physician's Orders** tab and review the orders for Tuesday at 1230.

13. Which of the orders listed below are nursing interventions? Select all that apply.

    _____ Temperature, pulse, respirations daily only

    _____ Finger-stick capillary glucose at bedtime tonight

    _____ Fasting blood glucose Wednesday morning

    _____ Continue blood pressure check every 8 hours

- Click the **Consultations** tab and review the data.

14. Why are multiple disciplines consulted to provide care for a patient?

15. What consultations have been made so far in William Jefferson's care?

16. Using critical thinking and based on William Jefferson's information, which nursing intervention should be the priority?
   a. Reinforce diet teaching regarding diabetic diet
   b. Assist patient to stand to void to improve bladder emptying
   c. Teach Mrs. Jefferson how to monitor Mr. Jefferson's blood glucose
   d. Involve Mr. Jefferson in card games to reduce boredom and agitation

17. Which statement reflects the evaluation phase in the plan of care for William Jefferson?
   a. Patient has a previous history of falls
   b. Instruct patient to call before getting up from bed
   c. Patient has experienced no falls during hospitalization
   d. Patient will remain free from injuries during hospitalization

LESSON 3

Patient Mobility

Reading Assignment: Body Mechanics and Patient Mobility (Chapter 8)

Patient: Kathryn Doyle, Room 503

Objectives:

1. List the complications associated with immobility.
2. Identify the responsibilities of the nurse concerning documentation of patient ambulation activities.
3. Recognize nursing diagnoses for the patient faced with mobility concerns.
4. Discuss the use of range-of-motion exercises.

Exercise 1

Writing Activity

15 minutes

1. When a patient with immobility concerns ambulates, what should the nurse monitor and document?

2. Identify common complications associated with immobility. (*Hint:* See Box 8-2 in your textbook.)

3. Listed below are interventions that must be taken when the nurse is assisting a patient who faints or collapses during ambulation. Match the columns to show the correct order of the interventions.

Intervention	Order of Priority
_____ Call for assistance.	a. First
_____ Document the event.	b. Second
_____ Stand with feet apart and back straight.	c. Third
_____ Assist the patient back to bed.	d. Fourth
_____ Quickly bring the patient close to your body.	e. Fifth
_____ Lower the patient to the floor.	f. Sixth

4. Match each position with its correct description.

Position	**Description**
_____ Semi-Fowler's	a. Lying with the head lowered and the body and legs on an incline plane
_____ Orthopneic	
	b. Lying on the back with the head of the bed elevated approximately 30 degrees
_____ Sims'	
_____ Prone	c. Kneeling with the body weight supported by the knees and chest
_____ Lithotomy	
	d. Lying face-down in a horizontal position
_____ Trendelenburg	
	e. Side-lying with the knee and thigh drawn upward toward the chest
_____ Genupectoral	
	f. Sitting up at a 90-degree angle; may be supported by a pillow on the overbed table
	g. Lying supine with hips and knees flexed; thighs abducted and rotated externally

5. What are range-of-motion exercises? Who is responsible for performing them?

6. Match each range-of-motion movement with its correct description.

Movement	**Description**
_____ Circumduction	a. Movement of the foot with the toes pointed upward
_____ External rotation	b. Movement of an extremity toward the midline of the body
_____ Dorsiflexion	c. Turning of the foot and leg away from the other leg
_____ Adduction	d. Movement of an extremity away from the midline of the body
_____ Abduction	e. Movement of the arm or leg in a full circle

7. _____ Sunlight influences the rate of bone loss. (True/False)

8. When preparing to lift, what should be included in the nurse's body mechanics? Select all that apply.

_____ Tuck chin downward

_____ Tilt pelvis slightly back

_____ Slightly flex knees

_____ Stand with feet slightly more than shoulder width apart

_____ Balance weight equally on both feet

Exercise 2

Virtual Hospital Activity

45 minutes

- Sign in to work at Pacific View Regional Hospital for Period of Care 2. (*Note:* If you are already in the Virtual Hospital from a previous exercise, click on **Leave the Floor** and then **Restart the Program** to get to the sign-in window.)
- From the Patient List, select Kathryn Doyle (Room 503).
- Click **Get Report** and read the Clinical Report.
- Click **Go to Nurses' Station**.
- Click **Chart** and then **503** to view Kathryn Doyle's chart.
- Review the information in the **History and Physical**, **Nursing Admission**, **Physician's Notes**, and **Physician's Orders** tabs.

1. What is Kathryn Doyle's primary medical diagnosis?

2. List Kathryn Doyle's other medical concerns.

3. What activity orders have been given by the physician?

- Click **Return to Nurses' Station** and then on **503** at the bottom of the screen to go to the patient's room.
- Read the **Initial Observations**.
- Click **Take Vital Signs** and review the information given.
- Click **Patient Care** and perform a head-to-toe assessment.

4. When faced with getting up and ambulating to the dining room, how does Kathryn Doyle respond?

5. When assisting Kathryn Doyle to ambulate, which instructions should be given to her when she feels weak?
   a. "Close your eyes until you get your bearings."
   b. "Point your head downward when you feel dizzy."
   c. "Take slow, deep breaths."
   d. "To increase oxygenation, breathe rapidly."

6. What factors in Kathryn Doyle's medical history may be further complicated by her continued immobility?

7. Based on the assessment, are there any reasons that she is unable to ambulate?

8. Given her refusal to ambulate and the physician's orders requiring her to do so, what should the nurse do?

9. Kathryn Doyle should be repositioned every _____ hours.

10. Kathryn Doyle has a wedge-shaped pillow between her legs. What purpose does this serve?

11. Based on the assessment and on diagnostic radiologic findings, is Kathryn Doyle experiencing any of the complications associated with immobility? If so, which?

- Click **Chart** and then **503** to view Kathryn Doyle's chart.
- Click the **Consultations** tab and review the information given.

12. What consultations have been made to improve or increase Kathryn Doyle's mobility?

13. What assistive device has been used to try to increase the patient's mobility?

14. Kathryn Doyle has a walker. What can be done to increase its stability?

15. Which actions are the nurse's responsibility concerning Kathryn Doyle's assistive devices? Select all that apply.

_____ The nurse should perform an assessment to confirm that the devices are being appropriately used.

_____ The nurse should remove the assistive devices for small periods each day to increase the patient's independence.

_____ The nurse must be present whenever the patient uses the assistive devices.

_____ The patient's permanent record must have evidence of the actions that have been selected from this list up to this point (assessment of use, removal of device, presence during use).

_____ The patient should be taught the appropriate use of the devices.

_____ The devices should be evaluated to ensure they are in working order.

16. During physical therapy, how much assistance does Kathryn Doyle need when ambulating?

17. What is being done in the physical therapy department to increase her lower body physical strength?

18. What special considerations are needed for Kathryn Doyle with regard to range-of-motion exercises because of her age?

19. Which two nursing diagnoses should the LPN/VN recognize as the priorities relating to Kathryn Doyle's mobility status?

Patient Safety

Reading Assignment: Safety (Chapter 10)

Patient: Kathryn Doyle, Room 503

Objectives:

1. Discuss safety factors related to advancing age.
2. Identify factors related to hospitalization that increase the risk for falls.
3. Discuss nursing interventions that reduce the safety risk for the hospitalized patient.
4. Recognize priority nursing diagnoses related to patient safety.

Exercise 1

Writing Activity

15 minutes

1. When using a gait belt to assist with ambulation, which are appropriate techniques? Select all that apply.

   _____ The gait belt should fit loosely around the hips.

   _____ The gait belt should be removed or loosened after use.

   _____ Walk behind the patient with the belt in hand to prevent falls.

   _____ Walk beside the patient with one arm around the waist and the other hand on the belt.

   _____ Walk on the weaker side of the patient.

   _____ Resist allowing the patient to rest on your arm.

2. What safety-related risk factors increase with age?

3. List several physiologic changes that may contribute to older adults' risk for injury.

4. What variables associated with hospitalization may increase a patient's risk for falls?

5. Which medication classifications can pose safety risks for older adult patients? Select all that apply.

_____ Vitamins

_____ Diuretics

_____ Hypnotics

_____ Antibiotics

_____ Antihistamines

6. Indicate whether each of the following statements is true or false.

a. _____ Nurses should use restraint devices whenever a patient is at risk for falls.

b. _____ Special interventions should be implemented to accommodate a patient with a visual disorder.

7. The national organization that provides guidelines to help reduce safety hazards in the workplace is

called the _____.

Exercise 2

Virtual Hospital Activity

45 minutes

• Sign in to work at Pacific View Regional Hospital for Period of Care 2. (*Note:* If you are already in the virtual hospital from a previous exercise, click on **Leave the Floor** and then **Restart the Program** to get to the sign-in window.)
• From the Patient List, select Kathryn Doyle (Room 503).
• Click **Get Report** and read the Clinical Report.
• Click **Go to Nurses' Station** and then click **503** at the bottom of the screen to enter the patient's room.
• Read the **Initial Observations**.
• Click **Check Armband** and then click **Take Vital Signs**.
• Click **Patient Care** and perform a head-to-toe assessment of Kathryn Doyle.

1. Use the assessment in the textbook and the factors below to determine Kathryn Doyle's fall risk. Select all that apply.

_____ History of seizures or fainting

_____ Older than age 70

_____ Recent falls

_____ Language barrier, loss of hearing

_____ Confused or disoriented

_____ History of drug and/or alcohol abuse

_____ Receiving multiple medications (such as tranquilizers, narcotics, hypnotics)

_____ New disability

_____ Neurologic problems

_____ Cardiovascular problems

_____ Overly independent attitude of patient and/or family

_____ Poor eyesight

_____ Urinary and/or bowel urgency

2. Based on your findings, Kathryn Doyle has _____ factors that increase her risk for falling.

3. _____ Kathryn Doyle's score places her in the "fall-prone" category. (True/False)

4. When performing an environmental assessment for Kathryn Doyle, which factors should be included in the assessment?

_____ Pathways to the bathroom, door, and closet

_____ Patient's emotional well-being

_____ Availability of operational call light

_____ Family's understanding of the plan of care

_____ Patient's knowledge of the unit routine

- Click **Chart** and then **503** to open Kathryn Doyle's chart.
- Click **Physician's Orders** and review the medications ordered for Kathryn Doyle.
- Click **Return to Nurses' Station**. Then click **Drug** in the bottom left corner of the screen. Use the Drug Guide to research the medications ordered for Kathryn Doyle.

5. Which of Kathryn Doyle's prescribed medications may increase her risk for injury? Select all that apply.

_____ Acetaminophen

_____ Oxycodone

_____ Ibuprofen

_____ Ferrous sulfate

_____ Calcium citrate

6. If the medications discussed in the previous question are administered to the patient, which special precautions should be taken? Select all that apply.

_____ Use restraints as indicated by nursing judgment.

_____ Assess toileting needs at least every 2 hours.

_____ Educate patient concerning medication side effects.

_____ Instruct patient on use of call light.

_____ Remind patient to call for assistance before getting up.

- Now click the **Laboratory Reports** and **Diagnostic Reports** tabs. Review each section.

7. Have any tests been performed that may provide information concerning the safety risks for Kathryn Doyle?

- Click the **History and Physical** and review the data provided.

8. What data did you find in the health history that may be used to assess Kathryn Doyle's safety risks?

9. When is the use of safety reminder devices (SRDs) indicated?

10. _____ It is appropriate to use an SRD to restrain an extremity for IV therapy. (True/False)

11. What complications may arise with the use of SRDs?

12. To avoid complications when using SRDs, what interventions should be used?

13. List techniques that may be used to avoid the need of SRDs.

14. Which two nursing diagnoses have the highest priority related to safety for Kathryn Doyle?

LESSON 5 ———————————————————

Assessment of Vital Signs

———————————————————————————

Reading Assignment: Vital Signs (Chapter 12)

Patient: Kathryn Doyle, Room 503

Objectives:

1. Recognize abnormal vital sign readings.
2. List the factors that will affect vital sign readings.
3. Discuss the actions that should be taken when abnormal readings are observed.
4. Discuss the use of pharmacologic agents in the management of febrile states.

Exercise 1

Writing Activity

15 minutes

1. List several factors that can cause an elevation in temperature.

2. A patient experiencing a dysfunction of what part of the brain may experience issues with thermoregulation?
   a. Hypothalamus
   b. Cerebellum
   c. Cerebral cortex
   d. Medulla

3. When planning care for a hospitalized patient, the nurse correctly recognizes that which times of day are associated with elevations in body temperature?
   a. 0600 to 0800
   b. 0800 to 1000
   c. 1400 to 1600
   d. 1600 to 1800

4. When describing a patient with an elevated temperature, which terms are appropriate to use? Select all that apply.

   _____ Afebrile

   _____ Hyposmia

   _____ Febrile

   _____ Hyperthermic

   _____ Pyretic

5. List several signs and symptoms that may accompany an elevated temperature. (*Hint:* See Box 12-5 in your textbook.)

6. _____ The metabolic rate will increase if the body's temperature is elevated. (True/False)

7. In addition to an elevated temperature, what other factors may affect the pulse rate? (*Hint:* See Box 12-9 in your textbook.)

8. The nurse is reviewing the patient's medical record and notes the patient has been experiencing an elevation in heart rate. What term will be used for this phenomenon?
   a. Tachycardia
   b. Tachypnea
   c. Transient hyper-pulse activity
   d. Bradycardia

Exercise 2

Virtual Hospital Activity

45 minutes

- Sign in to work at Pacific View Regional Hospital for Period of Care 1. (*Note:* If you are already in the virtual hospital from a previous exercise, click on **Leave the Floor** and then **Restart the Program** to get to the sign-in window.)
- From the Patient List, select Kathryn Doyle (Room 503).
- Click **Get Report** and read the Clinical Report.
- Click **Go to Nurses' Station**.
- Click **503** at the bottom of the screen to enter the patient's room.
- Click **Take Vital Signs**.

1. What are Kathryn Doyle's vital signs?

   T:

   BP:

   HR:

   RR:

2. Discuss any abnormal findings in the above vital signs.

3. Review Kathryn Doyle's list of prescribed medications. Are there any medications that may have resulted in elevations of her heart rate?
   a. Yes
   b. No

4. Based on your knowledge of Kathryn Doyle's health history, to what might her elevated temperature be attributed?

5. What interventions may be used to treat Kathryn Doyle's temperature elevation?

6. _____ Kathryn Doyle's temperature is elevated. This will commonly result in a decrease in heart rate. (True/False)

7. In addition to "routine" vital signs, when should the nurse assess vital signs for Kathryn Doyle?

    _____ After administering medication intended to lower the temperature.

    _____ Before administering medication intended to lower the temperature.

    _____ Before discharge from the skilled nursing facility.

    _____ In a skilled nursing facility there is no reason to assess additional vital signs.

    _____ If Kathryn Doyle comments, "I feel different."

8. The characteristics of Kathryn Doyle's temperature readings can best be described using which term?
    a. Fleeting
    b. Constant
    c. Intermittent
    d. Remittent

• Click on **Patient Care** and then **Nurse-Client Interactions**.
• Select and view the video titled **0730: Assessment—Biopsychosocial**. (*Note:* Check the virtual clock to see whether enough time has elapsed. You can use the fast-forward feature to advance the time by 2-minute intervals if the video is not yet available. Then click again on **Patient Care** and **Nurse-Client Interactions** to refresh the screen.)

9. In the video, what does Kathryn Doyle say or do to support the elevated temperature finding?

10. Discuss the impact that Kathryn Doyle's elevated temperature will have on the frequency of her assessments.

11. Which actions should the nurse take before reporting the elevation in Kathryn Doyle's temperature? Select all that apply.

    _____ Recheck the temperature to ensure proper functioning of equipment.

    _____ Administer acetaminophen.

    _____ Check the physician's orders to determine whether all orders have been posted.

    _____ Ask a nursing assistant to recheck the temperature.

    _____ Ask the patient whether she has eaten just before taking her temperature.

    _____ Give the patient a tepid sponge bath.

    _____ Administer ordered antibiotics.

- Click on **Patient Care**.
- Complete an assessment of Kathryn Doyle's chest and lower extremities.

12. The vascular assessment reveals pedal pulses 2+ bilaterally. Which term best describes this finding? (*Hint:* See Table 12-3 in your textbook.)
    a. Thready pulse
    b. Weak pulse
    c. Normal pulse
    d. Bounding pulse

- Click **Chart** and then **503** to view Kathryn Doyle's chart.
- Click the **Physician's Orders** tab and review the orders.

13. What orders has the physician left regarding Kathryn Doyle's temperature?

14. Before administering acetaminophen, the nurse should take what action(s)?

15. Which of Kathryn Doyle's prescribed medications may have had an impact on her current temperature? Select all that apply.

_____ Ferrous sulfate

_____ Calcium citrate

_____ Ibuprofen

_____ Docusate sodium

_____ Oxycodone

_____ Acetaminophen

- Click **Return to Room 503**.
- Click the **Drug** icon and review the information for acetaminophen.

16. How will acetaminophen reduce Kathryn Doyle's temperature?

17. When should Kathryn Doyle's temperature be retaken after she is given acetaminophen? Why?

18. Identify two priority nursing diagnoses that would be applicable to Kathryn Doyle's health status and her abnormal vital signs.

The Nursing Assessment

Reading Assignment: Physical Assessment (Chapter 13)

Patient: William Jefferson, Room 501

Objectives:

1. Discuss the role and importance of the shift report.
2. Discuss the assessment techniques that may be used when performing a physical assessment.
3. Review the two techniques that may be used to perform a comprehensive nursing assessment.
4. Identify abnormal findings on a physical examination.

Exercise 1

Writing Activity

15 minutes

1. Which are considered objective signs? Select all that apply.

   _____ The patient states, "I've never been this nauseated."

   _____ The patient is rubbing her abdomen and is grimacing.

   _____ The patient's pulse rate is 112 and is thready.

   _____ The patient states, "My left arm is itching a lot."

   _____ The patient has dark circles under her eyes.

   _____ The patient's skin is pale and diaphoretic.

   _____ The patient states, "I think I'm having a heart attack."

   _____ The patient's wound has purulent drainage.

2. Which questions should be included in an assessment of the patient's environmental risk factors? Select all that apply.

   _____ "How much alcohol do you drink in one day?"

   _____ "Do you have a place to stay when the temperature is below freezing?"

   _____ "Do you feel safe when walking in your neighborhood?"

   _____ "How long have you been smoking marijuana?"

   _____ "Does anyone in your family have diabetes?"

   _____ "Has asbestos been eliminated from your factory?"

   _____ "Do you use a space heater in your bedroom on cold nights?"

3. List some ways the nurse can enhance communication during a patient interview.

4. What should the nurse include when reviewing the patient's respiratory system?

5. What is the purpose of the nursing assessment?

6. What environmental considerations should be included in the physical assessment?

7. Discuss the approach you should take when planning to perform an assessment on a patient.

8. What are the two approaches used to perform a comprehensive nursing assessment?

9. Match each assessment technique with its corresponding definition. (*Hint:* See Box 12-4 in your textbook.)

Assessment Technique	Definition
_____ Inspection	a. The use of the fingertips to tap the body's surface and produce vibration and sound
_____ Palpation	b. A visual observation of the patient's body, responses to questioning, and nonverbal behaviors
_____ Auscultation	c. The use of the hands and sense of touch to gather information
_____ Percussion	d. The process of listening to sounds produced by the body

10. Match each assessment area with the position best used to assess it.

Assessment Area	Position
_____ Supine	a. Female genitalia
_____ Dorsal recumbent	b. Rectum and vagina
_____ Lithotomy	c. Head and neck, anterior thorax, and lungs
_____ Sims	d. Abdomen
_____ Lateral recumbent	e. Detection of heart murmurs

Exercise 2

Virtual Hospital Activity

45 minutes

- Sign in to work at Pacific View Regional Hospital for Period of Care 2. (*Note:* If you are already in the virtual hospital from a previous exercise, click on **Leave the Floor** and then **Restart the Program** to get to the sign-in window.)
- From the Patient List, select William Jefferson (Room 501).
- Click **Get Report** and read the Clinical Report.
- Click **Go to Nurses' Station**.
- Click **501** at the bottom of the screen to go to the patient's room. Inside the room, click **Patient Care**.

1. Which manner of data collection is being used by the nurse to assess William Jefferson?

- Click **Head & Neck** and review the assessment data in each area.

2. What tools are needed to complete this assessment? (*Hint:* See Figure 13-1 in your textbook.)

3. List any abnormal findings in the nurse's assessment of William Jefferson's head and neck.

4. What clues can be obtained from the examination of a patient's mouth and teeth?

5. What acronym is used to indicate that the patient's pupils are equal, round, and reactive to light and accomodation?

- Click **Chest** and review the assessment data in each area.

6. List any abnormal findings in the nurse's assessment of William Jefferson's chest.

7. Match each type of adventitious lung sound with its description.

Lung Sound	Description of Sound
_____ Crackles	a. Sound produced by a narrowing in the airway passages
_____ Wheezes	b. A bubbling sound that may be evidenced on inspiration
_____ Pleural friction rubs	c. Sound produced by inflammation in the pleural sac; may be a rubbing, grating, or friction sound

8. Heart sounds should be assessed for _____ and _____.

• Click **Back & Spine** and review the assessment data in each area.

9. List any abnormal findings in the nurse's assessment of William Jefferson's back and spine.

• Click **Upper Extremities** and review the assessment data in each area.

10. Identify any unusual findings in the assessment of the patient's upper extremities.

11. During an assessment of the abdomen, the patient's knees should be

    _____.

12. Which of the following is the *optimal* positioning of a patient while completing an abdominal assessment? (*Hint:* See Table 13-2 in your textbook.)
    a. Supine
    b. Prone
    c. Trendelenburg

13. Match the columns to show the appropriate order of actions for assessing a patient's abdomen.

Action	Order
_____ Auscultate for bowel sounds in each of the four quadrants.	a. First
_____ Palpate for masses or other abnormalities.	b. Second
_____ Visually inspect the abdomen for size, symmetry, and general appearance.	c. Third

• Click **Lower Extremities** and review the assessment data in each area.

14. List any findings of interest in the assessment of William Jefferson's lower extremities.

15. How is the capillary refill test performed?

16. William Jefferson's capillary refill is noted to be sluggish. What are potential causes of this finding?

Care of the Surgical Wound

Reading Assignment: Surgical Wound Care (Chapter 22)

Patient: Kathryn Doyle, Room 503

Objectives:

1. Define key terms associated with impaired wound healing.
2. Identify priorities in nursing diagnoses appropriate for the postoperative patient.
3. Discuss the phases of wound healing.
4. Identify potential complications related to wound healing.

Exercise 1

Writing Activity

15 minutes

1. Match each phase of wound healing with its correct definition.

   Phase of
   Wound Healing   **Definition**

   _____ Maturation   a. New cells are produced to fill the wound. This process closes the
                                          wound and aids in prevention of wound contamination.

   _____ Hemostasis
                                       b. Fibroblasts exit the wound and the wound continues to gain
   _____ Reconstruction   strength.

                                       c. Collagen is formed and the wound begins to develop a scar.

   _____ Inflammatory
                                       d. This phase begins at the time of the surgery. Blood products
                                          adhere to the site of the wound and begin to reduce blood loss.

2. There are several types of wound drainage. For each description of drainage given below, provide the
   type of fluid associated with it. (*Hint:* See Table 22-2 in your textbook.)

   a. Clear, watery fluid: _____

   b. Drainage containing blood: _____

   c. Thin, watery drainage containing blood: _____

   d. Thick, yellow, green, tan, or brown: _____

3. Listed below are terms associated with wound complications. Match each term with its definition.

Term	Definition
_____ Abscess	a. Passage of escape into the tissues, usually of blood, serum, or lymph
_____ Adhesion	b. Infection of the skin characterized by heat, pain, erythema, and edema
_____ Cellulitis	
_____ Dehiscence	c. Collection of extravasated blood trapped in the tissues or in an organ, resulting from incomplete hemostasis after surgery
_____ Evisceration	d. Cavity containing pus and surrounded by inflamed tissue, formed as a result of suppuration in a localized infection
_____ Extravasation	
_____ Hematoma	e. Protrusion of an internal organ through a wound or surgical incision
	f. Band of scar tissue that binds together two anatomic surfaces normally separated; most commonly found in the abdomen
	g. Separation of a surgical incision or rupture of a wound closure

4. Identify the three most common wound complications.

5. What physical findings at a wound site would indicate impaired healing?

6. _____ The majority of wound infections are evident by the time of discharge. (True/False)

7. List several patient factors that may affect postoperative wound healing.

Exercise 2

Virtual Hospital Activity

45 minutes

- Sign in to work at Pacific View Regional Hospital for Period of Care 1. (*Note:* If you are already in the virtual hospital from a previous exercise, click on **Leave the Floor** and then **Restart the Program** to get to the sign-in window.)
- From the Patient List, select Kathryn Doyle (Room 503).
- Click **Get Report** and read the Clinical Report.
- Click **Go to Nurses' Station**.
- Click **Chart** and then **503** to view Kathryn Doyle's chart.
- Click the **Nursing Admission** tab and review the report.

1. What was the reason for Kathryn Doyle's admission?

2. What surgical procedure did Kathryn Doyle undergo?

- Click the **History and Physical** tab and review the report.

3. What complications have necessitated Kathryn Doyle's continued hospitalization?

4. Discuss the link between Kathryn Doyle's anemia and the wound infection. (*Hint:* See Table 22-1 in your textbook.)

- Click **Return to Nurses' Station** and then click **503** at the bottom of the screen to go to the patient's room.
- Click **Patient Care** and complete a head-to-toe physical assessment.

5. Discuss the findings most pertinent to Kathryn Doyle's postoperative recovery.

- Click **Chart** and then click **503** to view Kathryn Doyle's chart.
- Once again, click the **Nursing Admission** tab and review the information provided.

6. What patient factors are most likely affecting Kathryn Doyle's prolonged recovery?

7. When planning Kathryn Doyle's diet, which of the following elements will help to promote wound healing? (*Hint:* See Table 22-1 in your textbook.)

_____ High protein

_____ High carbohydrates

_____ Vitamin C

_____ Vitamin A

_____ Vitamin D

8. When planning meals for Kathryn Doyle, which selections indicate an understanding of foods that are rich in vitamin C? Select all that apply. (*Hint:* Refer to Chapter 19 in your textbook if needed.)

_____ Orange juice

_____ Lean meat

_____ Kale salad

_____ Summer squash

_____ Bananas

9. _____ Leaving a wound open to air increases atmospheric oxygen to the wound, thus promoting healing. (True/False)

10. As discussed earlier, the wound may have drainage during the early postoperative period. What causes this drainage? Does it indicate a problem?

11. Identify three priorities in nursing diagnoses for Kathryn Doyle relating to her postoperative period.

12. Develop two positive patient outcomes for Kathryn Doyle.

13. Identify two areas that should be included in the teaching plan for Kathryn Doyle.

Pain Management

Reading Assignment: Pain Management, Comfort, Rest, and Sleep (Chapter 21)

Patient: Kathryn Doyle, Room 503

Objectives:

1. Identify the elements that must be included in an assessment of pain.
2. List medications used in the management of pain.
3. Relate the types or classifications of analgesics with the level of pain they are intended to treat.
4. Provide the appropriate patient education to accompany the administration of analgesics.

Exercise 1

Writing Activity

15 minutes

1. Identify several behavioral cues that may be associated with the presence of pain. (*Hint:* See Box 21-1 in your textbook.)

2. When caring for a patient in pain, which physiologic signs may be noted? Select all that apply. (*Hint:* See Box 21-3 in your textbook.)

_____ Hyperthermia

_____ Tachycardia

_____ Bradycardia

_____ Pallor

_____ Diaphoresis

_____ Constricted pupils

_____ Nausea

3. For what types of pain are nonopioids usually prescribed?

4. For what types of pain are opioids normally prescribed?

5. What should the nurse tell a patient who voices concerns about becoming addicted to opioid-containing medications?

6. The physician has ordered a TENS unit for a patient experiencing back pain. When discussing the device with the patient, what information should be included? Select all that apply.

_____ The device works by numbing pain receptors with the vibrations.

_____ The TENS unit provides mild electrical currents.

_____ The TENS unit is indicated for short-term use only.

_____ It is believed that endorphins are released by the TENS unit, aiding in pain relief.

_____ The TENS unit works to block pain impulses.

7. When administering NSAID medications, it is important that the nurse understand what information? Select all that apply.

_____ The risk for gastric toxicity from NSAIDs is greater in older adults than in younger adults.

_____ The maximum recommended dosage for acetaminophen is 4000 mg in a 24-hour period.

_____ NSAIDs are effective in the management of moderate pain.

_____ NSAIDs are associated with gastrointestinal bleeding.

_____ NSAIDs are available with a prescription only.

8. Which issues are associated with the undertreatment of pain by health care providers? Select all that apply.

_____ Concerns about the cost of medications prescribed

_____ Inadequate information about the drugs ordered

_____ Anxiety about potential patient injuries suffered while being medicated

_____ Laziness of the health care provider

_____ Concerns about fostering an addiction

_____ Safety issues

9. _____ is felt at a site other than the injured or diseased organ or part of the body.

Exercise 2

Virtual Hospital Activity

45 minutes

- Sign in to work at Pacific View Regional Hospital for Period of Care 1. (*Note:* If you are already in the virtual hospital from a previous exercise, click on **Leave the Floor** and then **Restart the Program** to get to the sign-in window.)
- From the Patient List, select Karen Doyle (Room 503).
- Click **Get Report** and read the Clinical Report.
- Click **Go to Nurses' Station** and then click **503** at the bottom of the screen to enter the patient's room.
- Read the **Initial Observations**.
- Click **Take Vital Signs**.

1. How does Kathryn Doyle describe her pain?

- Click **Chart** and then **503** to view Kathryn Doyle's chart.
- Click the **History and Physical** tab and review the report.

2. Review the reason for Kathryn Doyle's continued hospitalization.

- Click **Return to Room 503**.
- Click **MAR** and then tab **503** to view Kathryn Doyle's Medication Administration Record.
- Review the medications prescribed.
- Click **Return to Room 503**.
- Click the **Drug** icon at the bottom of the screen to review the drug resource guide.

3. Which medications have been prescribed for Kathryn Doyle to help reduce her pain? Select all that apply.

_____   Calcium citrate

_____   Oxycodone

_____   Ibuprofen

_____   Ferrous sulfate

_____   Docusate sodium

_____   Acetaminophen

4. For each medication you selected in the previous question, indicate whether it has been ordered on a scheduled or prn basis. Explain why each drug has been ordered.

5. Identify the classifications of each of the medications identified in the preceding questions.

6. What special considerations should be evaluated when administering pain medications to Kathryn Doyle?

7. What best explains the rationale for ibuprofen being prescribed on a scheduled basis rather than prn basis?
   a. Ibuprofen can also reduce the risk for infection and can be beneficial to the postoperative patient.
   b. Ibuprofen has antiinflammatory properties that aid the surgical patient in the recovery process.
   c. Ibuprofen is stronger than the other ordered analgesic medications and is more necessary to her recovery.
   d. The administration of ibuprofen on a set schedule will help to keep the patient's temperature reduced.

8. When administering oxycodone, the nurse is aware that which are potential side effects of the medication? Select all that apply.

   _____ Drowsiness

   _____ Nervousness

   _____ Agitation

   _____ Hypotension

   _____ Tachycardia

   _____ Anorexia

9. What should be assessed before the administration of oxycodone? Select all that apply.

_____   Time of last dosage

_____   Level of pain

_____   Vital signs

_____   Urinary output

_____   Reflexes

_____   Pupillary response

10. What patient education should be provided to Kathryn Doyle concerning oxycodone?

11. When administering oxycodone, the nurse should be aware that the duration of a dosage of the medication is what time period?
   a. 2 to 4 hours
   b. 3 to 6 hours
   c. 4 to 6 hours
   d. 5 to 7 hours

12. In addition to medication therapy, what nursing interventions may be implemented to reduce Kathryn Doyle's level of pain?

13. _____   Kathryn Doyle is suffering from chronic pain. (True/False)

LESSON 9

Nutritional Assessment in a Malnourished Patient

Reading Assignment: Nutritional Concepts and Related Therapies (Chapter 19)

Patient: Kathryn Doyle, Room 503

Objectives:

1. Identify the effects of nutritional status on postoperative recovery.
2. Define osteoporosis.
3. List the risk factors associated with the development of osteoporosis.
4. Discuss the role of the nurse in the promotion of healthy nutrition.

Exercise 1

Writing Activity

15 minutes

1. What is osteoporosis? What effects does this disorder have on the body?

2. Which factors contribute to the development of osteoporosis? Select all that apply.

   _____ Genetic influences

   _____ Physical activity

   _____ Gender

   _____ Large skeletal frame

   _____ Reduced intake of vitamin D, fluoride, and other trace minerals

   _____ Menopause

   _____ Smoking

3. Match each dietary nutrient with its correct definition.

Nutrient	**Definition**
_____ Complete proteins	a. Substances of plant origin that lack one or more of the essential amino acids
_____ Incomplete proteins	b. Organic compounds essential in small quantities for normal physiologic and metabolic functioning of the body
_____ Vitamins	
_____ Minerals	c. Inorganic compounds essential in small quantities for normal physiologic and metabolic functioning of the body
_____ Carbohydrates	d. Substances that are generally animal in nature and contain all nine essential amino acids
	e. Energy-producing organic compounds

4. How much sodium is needed daily by the older adult?
   a. 1200 mg
   b. 1300 mg
   c. 1500 mg
   d. 1600 mg

5. When planning a diet for the patient geared toward the prevention of osteoporosis, what items should be included? Select all that apply.

   _____ Soy milk

   _____ Kale

   _____ Pumpkin

   _____ Cheese

   _____ Cauliflower

6. In each blank in the list below, write "High" or "Low" to indicate the dietary factors that will reduce calcium loss in the urine.

   • _____-sodium diets

   • _____-potassium diets

   • _____-protein diets

7. Which are signs and symptoms of iron deficiency anemia? Select all that apply.

   _____ Enlarged thyroid gland

   _____ Fatigue

   _____ Susceptibility to tooth decay

   _____ Pale skin

   _____ Decreased zinc absorption

   _____ Headache

   _____ Apathy

8. When planning a diet for the patient with iron deficiency anemia, what foods should be included to increase iron intake? Select all that apply.

   _____ Salmon

   _____ Flounder

   _____ Broccoli

   _____ Legumes

   _____ Citrus fruits

9. Which factors can inhibit iron absorption? Select all that apply. (*Hint:* See Box 19-5 in your textbook.)

   _____ Some medications, such as antacids

   _____ Fish, meat, and poultry that contain MFP

   _____ Calcium in milk and supplements

   _____ Polyphenols, which are compounds found in coffee, tea, and red wine

   _____ Ascorbic acid (vitamin C) when ingested with iron-containing foods

10. Which factors can promote the absorption of iron? Select all that apply. (*Hint:* See Box 19-5 in your textbook.)

    _____ Ingestion of vitamin B_6

    _____ Meat and fish intake

    _____ Ingestion of citrus beverages

    _____ Taking the medication at bedtime

    _____ Taking the medication with a large glass of water

11. How do complete and incomplete proteins differ?

12. When caring for the patient on antihypertensive therapy, what supplementation is indicated?
    a. Thiamine
    b. Niacin
    c. Riboflavin
    d. Pyroxidine

Exercise 2

Virtual Hospital Activity

45 minutes

- Sign in to work at Pacific View Regional Hospital for Period of Care 3. (*Note:* If you are already in the virtual hospital from a previous exercise, click on **Leave the Floor** and then **Restart the Program** to get to the sign-in window.)
- From the Patient List, select Kathryn Doyle (Room 503).
- Click **Get Report** and read the Clinical Report.
- Click **Go to Nurses' Station** and then click **503** at the bottom of the screen to enter the patient's room.
- Read the **Initial Observations**.
- Click **Chart** and then **503** to view Kathryn Doyle's chart.
- Review the information within the **History and Physical**, **Nursing Admission**, and **Consultations** tabs.

1. What complications of Kathryn Doyle's surgery are reported in the History and Physical?

2. According to the consultations, what is the physician's impression concerning the nutritional status of this patient?

3. Which postoperative complications identified in question 1 of this exercise are further complicated by Kathryn Doyle's nutritional status? Why does her nutritional status have these effects?

4. What risk factors for the development of osteoporosis does Kathryn Doyle have?

5. Kathryn Doyle reports that she has lost 4 pounds in the last 5 months and has lost 15 pounds in the last 2 years. What psychosocial factors may have contributed to her weight loss?

6. What is one physical factor that may have contributed to her weight loss?

7. What are the impressions of the dietary consultation?

8. Discuss the plan outlined in the dietary consultation.

9. What role will the increased protein have in her diet?

10. Kathryn Doyle's physician has prescribed a soft diet. Which selections are appropriate for inclusion in her dietary plan? Select all that apply.

_____ Whole wheat toast

_____ Poached eggs

_____ Baked cod fish

_____ Broccoli casserole

_____ Fiber snack bars

_____ Rice

- Click **Physician's Orders** tab and review the information given.

11. What medications have been ordered to aid Kathryn Doyle in meeting the nutritional requirements of her body and health status?

- Click **Return to Room 503**.
- Click the **Drug** icon at the bottom of the screen and review the medications you identified in the previous question.

12. What are the nursing considerations that should be observed when administering each of these drugs?

- Click **Return to Room 503**.
- Read the **Initial Observations**.
- Click **Take Vital Signs** and review the results.
- Click **Patient Care** and perform a head-to-toe physical assessment.

13. What assessment findings are related to Kathryn Doyle's limited nutritional intake?

14. When assisting Kathryn Doyle to plan her dietary intake, the nurse recognizes that which of the following dietary nutrients will best enable her to increase her energy level?
    a. Fat
    b. Fiber
    c. Carbohydrate
    d. Protein

15. What positive effects will an increase in fluid intake have on Kathryn Doyle's assessment findings?

16. Kathryn Doyle's physician has prescribed calcium supplements. Vitamin D is needed to promote calcium absorption. Which are good sources of vitamin D? Select all that apply.

    _____ Sunlight exposure

    _____ Leafy green vegetables

    _____ Citrus fruits

    _____ Egg yolks

    _____ Liver

    _____ Whole grains

17. If Kathryn Doyle refuses to increase her intake, what noninvasive measures can the nurse take?

Nutritional Assessment in an Overweight Patient

Reading Assignment: Nutritional Concepts and Related Therapies (Chapter 19)

Patient: Delores Gallegos, Room 502

Objectives:

1. Identify the health risks that accompany obesity.
2. Calculate the caloric needs of a patient.
3. Discuss the impact of aging on caloric needs.
4. Discuss the relationship between diuretic therapy and nutritional needs.

Exercise 1

Writing Activity

30 minutes

1. How is obesity defined?

2. When measuring obesity, which factors are reviewed? Select all that apply.

   _____ Height

   _____ Weight

   _____ Age

   _____ Daily caloric intake

   _____ Presence of physiologic health conditions

3. List several health risks associated with obesity.

4. What interventions are available for the treatment of obesity?

5. Match each food with the fatty acid class to which it belongs.

Food	**Fatty Acid Class**
_____ Margarine	a. Saturated
_____ Corn oil	b. Monounsaturated
_____ Beef tallow	c. Polyunsaturated
_____ Egg yolk	d. Trans
_____ Coconut oil	
_____ Chicken fat	
_____ Most fish oils	
_____ Peanuts	
_____ Olives	

6. Potassium has several functions in the human body. Fill in the blanks in the following list describing the actions of potassium.

Potassium:

- Helps to regulate _____ and _____ within cells

- Promotes transmission of _____ impulses

- Aids in functioning of _____ muscles

- Assists in the regulation of _____ balance

7. Which foods are considered good sources of dietary potassium? Select all that apply.

_____ Fruits

_____ Leafy green vegetables

_____ Avocados

_____ Legumes

_____ Nuts

_____ Milk

_____ Potatoes

8. The feeling of fullness and satisfaction from ingestion of food is known as _____.

Exercise 2

Virtual Hospital Activity

30 minutes

- Sign in to work at Pacific View Regional Hospital for Period of Care 1. (*Note:* If you are already in the virtual hospital from a previous exercise, click on **Leave the Floor** and then **Restart the Program** to get to the sign-in window.)
- From the Patient List, select Delores Gallegos (Room 502).
- Click **Get Report** and read the Clinical Report.
- Click **Go to Nurses' Station** and then **Chart**.
- Click **502** to view Delores Gallegos' chart.
- Click and review the **History and Physical**, **Physician's Notes**, **Physician's Orders**, and **Nursing Admission** tabs.

1. How is Delores Gallegos' weight described in the physical exam section?

2. What effects has Delores Gallegos' weight had on her health status?

3. What other significant health history is identified?

4. What is Delores Gallegos' approximate BMI?
   a. 26
   b. 28
   c. 30
   d. 32

- Click **Return to Nurses' Station** and then **MAR**.
- Click tab **502** to view Delores Gallegos' Medication Administration Record.
- Click **Return to Nurses' Station**. Then click **Drug** in the bottom left corner of the screen. Use the Drug Guide to review the medications that have been ordered for the patient.

5. The following medications have been ordered for Delores Gallegos to treat her heart failure. Match each medication with its mechanism of action.

Medication	Mechanism of Action
_____ Furosemide	a. Slows heart rate; decreases blood pressure and cardiac output
_____ Captopril	b. Produces a diuretic effect
_____ Metoprolol	c. Improves cardiac output and increases exercise tolerance

6. When administering furosemide, the nurse must be aware that this drug is associated with increased excretion of which electrolytes? Select all that apply.

_____ Magnesium

_____ Calcium

_____ Sodium

_____ Potassium

_____ Chloride

7. What laboratory tests should be monitored when a patient is receiving diuretic therapy?

- Click **Return to Nurses' Station**.
- Click **Chart** and then **502** to view Delores Gallegos' chart.
- Click the **Laboratory Reports** tab and review the results given.

8. The normal value for potassium within the body is between _____ and _____ mEq/L.

9. How do Delores Gallegos' electrolytes in the laboratory results for Wednesday at 0600 compare with normal limits?

- Click **Return to Nurses' Station** and then click **502** at the bottom of the screen to enter Delores Gallegos' room.
- Click **Patient Care** and then **Nurse-Client Interactions**.
- Select and view the video titled **0730: Cultural Preferences**. (*Note:* Check the virtual clock to see whether enough time has elapsed. You can use the fast-forward feature to advance the time by 2-minute intervals if the video is not yet available. Then click again on **Patient Care** and **Nurse-Client Interactions** to refresh the screen.)

10. What is Delores Gallegos' chief complaint regarding her hospital diet?

11. What are the responsibilities of the nurse when faced with the dietary concerns voiced by Delores Gallegos?

12. How does culture affect dietary intake?

- Click **Check Armband** and review the information given.

13. What impact does Delores Gallegos' age have on her caloric needs?

14. What is the range of a healthy weight for Delores Gallegos? (*Hint:* See Figure 19-5.)
    a. 89 to 103 pounds
    b. 100 to 150 pounds
    c. 104 to 131 pounds
    d. 136 to 158 pounds

15. The dietary consultation is pending. What dietary recommendations would you anticipate for Delores Gallegos?

16. _____ Given Delores Gallegos' medical condition, she is not a good candidate for the DASH diet. (True/False)

11

Life Span Development

Reading Assignment: Life Span Development (Chapter 24)

Patient: Kathryn Doyle, Room 503

Objectives:

1. Identify role changes associated with aging.
2. Discuss the developmental tasks associated with older adults.
3. Define physiologic theories associated with aging.
4. Define the psychological theories associated with aging.

Exercise 1

Writing Activity

15 minutes

1. The nurse is reviewing data collected from a patient who has reported she is the lead decision maker in her household in regard to financial matters, child care, and home management. Her family unit can best be described using which term?
   a. Patriarchal
   b. Matriarchal
   c. Autocratic
   d. Democratic

2. Which statement concerning the needs of the aging adult is correct?
   a. Caloric needs will increase only slightly to meet the demands put on the body.
   b. Older adults generally sleep fewer hours per night as they age.
   c. The importance of relationships decreases after age 70.
   d. The intensity of sexual drives remains constant throughout the life span.

3. The body's response to aging includes which changes? Select all that apply. (*Hint:* See Table 24-4 in your textbook.)

   _____ Body weight increases until age 45 or 50.

   _____ The accumulation of adipose tissue in women is more pronounced in the waist, chest, and lower abdomen.

   _____ Saliva production increases.

   _____ Loss of height begins to occur after age 50.

   _____ There is a reduction in the perception of taste and smell.

   _____ An increase in basal metabolic rate is normal.

   _____ Tactile sensations decrease.

4. Indicate whether each of the following statements is true or false.

   a. _____ Necessary developmental skills in late adulthood include maximization of independence and the maintenance of a high level of involvement.

   b. _____ Older people are generally slower than younger people with regard to cognition but often are more accurate.

5. Older adults should maintain a daily fluid intake of _____ mL/day.

6. What are the chief determinants of an individual's psychological response to aging?

7. The age group known as "young older adult" includes people between the ages of _____ and _____.

8. A form of discrimination and prejudice against older adults is known as

_____.

9. Match each physiologic aging theory with its correct description.

Physiologic Aging Theory	**Description**
_____ Autoimmunity theory	a. Supports the belief that structural and functional changes associated with advancing age are increased by abuses on the body
_____ Free radical theory	
_____ Wear-and-tear theory	b. Supports the belief that the response to aging is determined by genetic connections
_____ Biologic programming theory	c. Supports the belief that the body is less able to recognize "self"; produces antibodies against itself
	d. Supports the belief that an accumulation of cellular waste promotes the aging process

10. Match each psychological aging theory with its correct definition.

Psychological Aging Theory	**Description**
_____ Disengagement theory	a. Links successful aging to the ability to maintain roles and activities
_____ Activity theory	b. The belief that aging individuals will remove themselves from other elements of society
_____ Continuity theory	c. The belief that older individuals with more social interaction have better personal adjustment

Exercise 2

Virtual Hospital Activity

45 minutes

- Sign in to work at Pacific View Regional Hospital for Period of Care 1. (*Note:* If you are already in the virtual hospital from a previous exercise, click on **Leave the Floor** and then **Restart the Program** to get to the sign-in window.)
- From the Patient List, select Kathryn Doyle (Room 503).
- Click **Get Report** and read the Clinical Report.
- Click **Go to Nurses' Station** and then click **503** at the bottom of the screen to enter the patient's room.
- Click **Check Armband** and review the information given.
- Click **Chart** and then click **503** to view Kathryn Doyle's chart.
- Click and review the notes in the **Nursing Admission**, **History and Physical**, and **Consultations** tabs.

1. How old is Kathryn Doyle?

2. Why was Kathryn Doyle initially admitted to the health care facility?

3. What age-related changes contributed to the injury experienced by Kathryn Doyle?

4. What are her primary psychosocial concerns?

5. What does Kathryn Doyle find stressful about her home life?

6. The Doyle household and its inhabitants are an example of a(n) _____ family.

7. Kathryn Doyle is at the _____ stage in the life cycle.

8. Discuss the role changes that Kathryn Doyle has encountered since the death of her spouse.

9. Kathryn Doyle is experiencing the Erikson stage of psychosocial development known as

   _____ versus _____.

10. What takes place during this stage?

11. Based on her responses in the Nursing Admission assessment, evaluate Kathryn Doyle's success in this stage of development.

12. List the developmental tasks for this stage of Kathryn Doyle's life. (*Hint:* See Box 24-21 in your textbook.)

13. _____ Kathryn Doyle is progressing successfully through the aging process as outlined by the activity theory of aging. (True/False)

14. Although there is support for the disengagement theory of aging, there is also criticism concerning its accuracy. The concerns relating to this theory include which of the following? Select all that apply.

_____ It does not allow for many active, functional older adults.

_____ There is little ability to apply this theory to both men and women.

_____ It is seen as biased against disabled seniors.

_____ The process is not seen in all cultural groups; thus it is not universal.

_____ It is somewhat pessimistic concerning the longevity of seniors and their abilities to remain contributing members of society.

15. According to Erikson, if Kathryn Doyle does not find satisfaction with her accomplishments, she will

    experience _____ and _____.

16. _____ Some widowed older adults in need of companionship will consider remarrying as a solution to the challenges presented by the death of a spouse. (True/False)

17. For Kathryn Doyle, acceptance of her own _____ and preparation for death is a task associated with late adulthood.

- Click **Return to Room 503**.
- Click **Patient Care** and complete an assessment of the head, neck, chest, and pelvis.

18. There are concerns about Kathryn Doyle's nutritional status. What assessment findings support these concerns? Select all that apply.

    _____ Status of oral mucosa

    _____ Affect

    _____ Cognition

    _____ Status of skin turgor

    _____ Sense of smell

    _____ Status of dentures

19. What care interventions can be implemented to improve the nutritional intake of Kathryn Doyle?

20. What urinary findings are noted that may be associated with aging?

21. What changes in the urinary system occur with aging that may be partially responsible for the assessment findings of Kathryn Doyle?

Establishment of End-of-Life Wishes

Reading Assignment: Loss, Grief, Dying, and Death (Chapter 25)

Patient: Goro Oishi, Room 505

Objectives:

1. Discuss the concepts of an advance directive.
2. Recognize priority nursing diagnoses needed by the family members of a dying patient.
3. Discuss the emotional support needed by the family members of a dying patient.
4. List potential referrals for the family experiencing an impending death.

Exercise 1

Writing Activity

15 minutes

1. The nurse is reviewing the document provided by a patient that outlines his health care wishes should he be unable to make decisions. What is the term used to refer to this document?
   a. An advance directive
   b. A power of attorney
   c. A guardianship
   d. A health care liaison

2. What is required to make the above document legal and binding? Select all that apply.

   _____ The document must be signed and dated by the patient.

   _____ The signing must be witnessed by two health care providers.

   _____ The document must be reviewed and approved by the physician.

   _____ The signing must be witnessed by two people who are not relatives of the patient.

   _____ The signing must be witnessed by two family members of the patient.

   _____ The patient must seek spiritual counseling before signing the document.

3. If aggressive technological options are not used on an older adult, what interventions should the nurse provide?

4. A document that directs medical treatment in accordance with a patient's wishes in the event of a terminal illness or condition is called a _____.

5. The designation of a person other than the patient to make health care decisions on the patient's behalf is called a _____.

6. In Bowlby's stages of mourning, which stage is considered the most distressful?
   a. Numbing
   b. Yearning and Searching
   c. Despair
   d. Disorganization

7. A patient has sought counseling for difficulty dealing with the loss of a parent more than a year ago. The patient reports that she is just not able to move forward and feel any better. This type of grief is best described as which type?
   a. Delayed grief
   b. Dysfunctional mourning
   c. Chronic grief
   d. Exaggerated grief

Exercise 2

Virtual Hospital Activity

45 minutes

- Sign in to work at Pacific View Regional Hospital for Period of Care 1. (*Note:* If you are already in the virtual hospital from a previous exercise, click on **Leave the Floor** and then **Restart the Program** to get to the sign-in window.)
- From the Patient List, select Goro Oishi (Room 505).
- Click **Get Report** and read the Clinical Report.
- Click **Go to Nurses' Station**.
- Click **Chart** and then **505** to view Goro Oishi's chart.
- Click the **History and Physical** tab and review the report.

1. Why was Goro Oishi admitted to the hospital? What is his current status?

2. What elements have been identified in Goro Oishi's plan of care according to his History and Physical?

- Click the **Physician's Notes** tab and read the progress notes.
- Click the **Consents** tab and review the information given.

3. Who is in control of Goro Oishi's medical care? Why is this person able to direct his care?

4. Which statement regarding the roles of those in charge of Goro Oishi's health care is correct?
   a. Mrs. Oishi will have the authority to handle her husband's financial affairs.
   b. Mrs. Oishi will be required to consult with the entire family to obtain a consensus when making critical decisions.
   c. The physician will be required to make the final determination regarding the health care decisions.
   d. The Oishi family attorney will be required to go to court to make Mrs. Oishi her husband's health care guardian.
   e. Mrs. Oishi can make all of the health care decisions for her husband in the event that he is unable to make decisions for himself.

5. What provisions have been made in case Mrs. Oishi is unable to accept the role?

6. In the event that Goro Oishi's family members do not agree with Mrs. Oishi's plans for his care, what will happen?
   a. Mrs. Oishi will be required to seek approval from the hospital's ethics committee to continue with her wishes.
   b. Mrs. Oishi will need to seek approval from a court of law to enforce her wishes regarding her husband's care.
   c. Mrs. Oishi can continue to have her wishes for her husband's care carried out.
   d. Mr. Oishi's physician will have the authority to determine which party's wishes concerning Mr. Oishi's care will be implemented.

7. List the specific powers given to Mrs. Oishi by the advance directive.

8. Which physician's order specifies what is to be done in the event Goro Oishi stops breathing?

9. List the health care decisions that were addressed by Goro Oishi's advance directive.

- Click the **Consultations** tab and review the information given.

10. What referrals have been made to assist the Oishi family at this time?

11. What was the outcome of this consultation?

- Click the **Nurse's Notes** tab and review the notes.

12. Discuss the family's support of Goro Oishi's health care directives.

13. Identify one goal and one outcome for the Oishi family during the dying process.

14. Identify a priority nursing diagnosis for the Oishi family during the dying process.

15. Consider the situation of Goro Oishi's son. Is his loss best considered to be situational loss or maturational loss?

Care of the Dying Patient

Reading Assignment: Loss, Grief, Dying, and Death (Chapter 25)

Patient: Goro Oishi, Room 505

Objectives:

1. Define palliative care.
2. List the priority needs of the dying patient.
3. Recognize the physiologic signs and symptoms of impending death.
4. List the clinical signs of death.
5. Identify nursing interventions in the care of the dying patient.

Exercise 1

Writing Activity

15 minutes

1. Identify the three most important needs of the dying patient.

2. _____ is the provision of care to promote comfort of a dying patient. Measures are not geared toward sustaining life.

3. When caring for the patient who is dying, what changes in vital signs signal impending death? Select all that apply.

_____ Weak pulse

_____ Thready pulse

_____ Sharp spikes of hypertensive episodes

_____ Shallow respirations

_____ Episodes of tachypnea

4. The nurse is caring for a patient who is nearing death. The patient seems restless. This is of concern to the family members, who question the nurse about this behavior. What response by the nurse is most appropriate?
   a. "Unfortunately, these behaviors are the result of air hunger."
   b. "The restless movements you are seeing are likely the result of some unrelieved discomfort."
   c. "As death nears, the body's levels of oxygen are diminished, resulting in these restless movements."
   d. "This is your loved one's last attempts to communicate."

5. List the clinical signs of death.

6. Which statements regarding the concept of death are correct for most adults between the ages of 45 and 65 years? Select all that apply. (*Hint:* See Table 25-1 in your textbook.)

_____ The adult fears a long and lingering death.

_____ The adult's attitudes concerning death are influenced by cultural beliefs.

_____ The adult believes that death will allow freedom from pain and a reunion with deceased family and friends.

_____ The adult accepts his or her own mortality.

_____ The adult experiences peaks of death anxiety.

Exercise 2

Virtual Hospital Activity

30 minutes

- Sign in to work at Pacific View Regional Hospital for Period of Care 1. (*Note:* If you are already in the virtual hospital from a previous exercise, click on **Leave the Floor** and then **Restart the Program** to get to the sign-in window.)
- From the Patient List, select Goro Oishi (Room 505).
- Click **Get Report** and read the Clinical Report.
- Click **Go to Nurses' Station** and then click **505** at the bottom of the screen to enter the patient's room.
- Read the **Initial Observations**.
- Click **Take Vital Signs**.

1. List Goro Oishi's vital signs.

BP:

T:

HR:

RR:

SpO$_2$:

- Click **Patient Care** and complete a physical assessment of Goro Oishi's **Head & Neck**.

2. Which findings in the head and neck assessment are consistent with Goro Oishi's comatose and brain-damaged status?

- Click **Chest** and complete a physical assessment.

3. What finding in the chest assessment supports the comatose diagnosis?

- Click on the remaining sections of the head-to-toe assessment and review the notes for each area.

4. What additional findings in the remainder of the assessment support the diagnosis?

5. Discuss Goro Oishi's urinary output.

- Click **Chart** and then **505** to view Goro Oishi's chart.
- Click the **Physician's Orders** tab and review the orders.

6. Several interventions have been ordered to promote Goro Oishi's level of comfort. For each rationale listed below, provide the intervention ordered. (*Note:* More than one word may be written in each blank.)

   - To assist with respiratory function and promote comfort, _____

     _____.

   - To aid in maintaining oxygenation and reduce respiratory distress, _____

     _____ has been ordered.

   - To reduce respiratory distress and choking potential, _____.

   - To decrease discomfort associated with drying of the mucous membranes, _____

     _____.

   - To reduce fever and promote comfort, administer _____.

   - To increase Goro Oishi's level of comfort, perform _____
     three times a day.

7. As noted, Goro Oishi has a DNR order in place. What is the purpose of the other orders concerning his care?

Exercise 3

Virtual Hospital Activity

15 minutes

- Sign in to work at Pacific View Regional Hospital for Period of Care 3. (*Note:* If you are already in the virtual hospital from the previous exercise, click on **Leave the Floor** and then **Restart the Program** to get to the sign-in window.)
- From the Patient List, select Goro Oishi (Room 505).
- Click **Get Report** and read the Clinical Report.
- Click **Go to Nurses' Station** and then click **505** at the bottom of the screen to enter the patient's room.
- Read the **Initial Observations**.

1. What physiologic changes occurred during the previous shift?

- Click **Take Vital Signs** and review the findings.

2. Describe the changes noted in the vital signs and the implications of each change.

- Click **Patient Care** and complete a physical assessment of Goro Oishi's **Head & Neck**.

3. What significant changes have taken place and are manifested in the assessment of the head and neck?

4. What findings indicate a reduction in the patient's cardiopulmonary functioning?

5. Identify the priority nursing diagnosis for the Oishi family during this period.

6. What care interventions to the family are appropriate at this time?

7. Goro Oishi's chart indicates that he is Buddhist. What cultural considerations may be indicated as he approaches death?
   a. Requests for the presence of an ordained monk or nun
   b. Requests to close the eyes
   c. Requests to accompany the body at all times including transport to the morgue and to the funeral home
   d. Requests to administer the sacraments of Penance

8. Identify five items that must be included in the nurse's documentation after Goro Oishi dies. (*Hint:* See Box 25-10 in your textbook.)

Health Promotion in the Older Adult

Reading Assignment: Health Promotion and Care of the Older Adult (Chapter 33)

Patient: Carlos Reyes, Room 504

Objectives:

1. Identify physiologic concerns associated with aging.
2. Identify physiologic changes associated with aging.
3. Identify psychosocial concerns associated with aging.
4. Recognize nursing interventions to promote the care of the older adult.

Exercise 1

Writing Activity

30 minutes

1. Older adults may face _____ and _____ regarding their changing roles within society and the family.

2. What interventions may be used to increase a patient's orientation to reality?

3. The progressive impairment of cognitive function is known as _____.

4. Which integumentary system changes are associated with aging? Select all that apply.

_____ An increase in the production of sebum

_____ An increase in bruising and susceptibility to trauma

_____ Reduction in perspiration

_____ Decreased wound healing time

_____ Increased susceptibility to infection

5. How are urinary and fecal incontinence related to aging?

6. Match each type of incontinence with its correct description.

Type of Incontinence	Description
_____ Stress urinary incontinence	a. Associated with central nervous system disorders; characterized by involuntary urine loss after a sudden urge to void
_____ Urge urinary incontinence	
_____ Functional urinary incontinence	b. Occurs as a result of an inability or unwillingness to toilet because of physical limitations or emotional issues
	c. Involuntary loss of a small amount of urine with increased abdominal pressure

7. Many changes take place in the respiratory system as a person ages. Fill in the blanks to complete the list of these age-related respiratory changes:

   • _____ and _____ of the thoracic cage

   • Reduced lung _____

   • _____ vital capacity

   • Reduced number and effectiveness of the lungs' _____

   • Reduced air _____ and secretions

8. Many changes also take place in the cardiovascular system as a person ages. Fill in the blanks to complete the list of these age-related cardiovascular changes:

   • Loss of structural _____

   • _____ and more _____ heart valves

   • Decrease in _____ cells and slowed electrical conduction

   • Possible decrease in heart rate

   • Reduced cardiac _____

   • Development of arteriosclerosis

   • Increased risk for _____

9. What nursing interventions may be used to reduce cardiovascular complications?

10. According to the American Medical Association, which are classifications of abuse? Select all that apply.

_____ Physical abuse

_____ Psychological abuse

_____ Behaviors of isolation

_____ Medical abuse

_____ Neglect

_____ Misuse of assets

11. Which statements concerning the use of medications in older adults are correct? Select all that apply.

_____ On average, the older adult takes up to 7 prescription medications.

_____ Laxatives and vitamin supplements are commonly used medications among older adults.

_____ The average older adult is currently taking 2 nonprescription medications.

_____ The use of multiple drugs may reduce the therapeutic benefits of the medications taken.

_____ Using more than one pharmacy to fill prescriptions will increase the risk factors associated with polypharmacy.

_____ The body's ability to absorb, transport, and eliminate medications is increased with age.

12. _____ Nearly 25% of people 70 years of age and older report falls each year. (True/False)

Exercise 2

Virtual Hospital Activity

30 minutes

- Sign in to work at Pacific View Regional Hospital for Period of Care 1. (*Note:* If you are already in the virtual hospital from a previous exercise, Click on **Leave the Floor** and then **Restart the Program** to get to the sign-in window.)
- From the Patient List, select Carlos Reyes (Room 504).
- Click **Get Report** and read the Clinical Report.
- Click **Go to Nurses' Station** and then click **504** at the bottom of the screen to enter the patient's room.
- Click **Check Armband** and then click **Take Vital Signs** and review the information given.
- Click **Patient Care** and complete a head-to-toe assessment.

1. How old is Carlos Reyes?

2. In what phase of adulthood is Carlos Reyes?

3. What changes associated with aging are noted in Carlos Reyes' skin?

4. What are the allergies listed for Carlos Reyes?

5. Discuss nursing interventions that may be used to compensate for hearing loss.

6. While assessing Carlos Reyes' lower extremities and looking at his feet, what age-related findings are noted?

7. List several abnormalities noted in the assessment of Carlos Reyes' upper extremities and abdomen.

8. What impact might nocturia have on Carlos Reyes' health status?

- Click **Chart** and then **504** to view Carlos Reyes' chart.
- Click the **History and Physical** tab and review the information provided.

9. Carlos Reyes was admitted to the hospital after experiencing a _____

   _____.

10. Which cardiovascular disease risk factors does Carlos Reyes have? Select all that apply.

_____ Age

_____ Lifestyle

_____ Hyperlipidemia

_____ Heredity

_____ Obesity

_____ Hypertension

11. Does Carlos Reyes have a history of any pulmonary complications/disorders?

12. According to the History and Physical, in addition to rehabilitation, why has Carlos Reyes been admitted to the Skilled Nursing Unit?

13. Consider Carlos Reyes' age. What diagnostic examinations are recommended to be performed annually? Select all that apply.

_____ Eye examination

_____ Physical examination

_____ Prostate examination

_____ Stool for occult blood examination

_____ Hearing examination

15

Basic Mental Health Nursing Concepts

Reading Assignment: Concepts of Mental Health (Chapter 34)

Patient: Carlos Reyes, Room 504

Objectives:

1. Discuss the evaluation of mental health along a continuum.
2. Identify factors that affect a patient's position on the mental health continuum.
3. Discuss the impact of hospitalization on mental health.
4. Discuss nursing interventions to reduce the stressors associated with hospitalization.

Exercise 1

Writing Activity

15 minutes

1. How is mental health defined?

2. What factors must be assessed to determine a patient's placement along the continuum?

3. Mental illness may be characterized by patterns of behavior that are _____,

   _____, or _____.

4. When considering the three elements of personality, which best describes the role of the id?
   a. Provides the moral conscious for actions
   b. Seeks to promote emotional homeostasis
   c. Aids in the perception of reality
   d. Strives for perfection

5. Match each commonly used defense mechanism with its correct description. (*Hint:* See Table 34-1 in your textbook.)

Defense Mechanism	Description
_____ Compensation	a. An avoidance of reality
_____ Conversion	b. The intentional exclusion of painful thoughts, experiences, or impulses
_____ Denial	
	c. Excelling in one area to make up for deficits in another area
_____ Displacement	
	d. Placing the blame for personal shortcomings on another person or group
_____ Identification	
_____ Projection	e. Turning emotional conflicts into a physical symptom
_____ Rationalization	f. A process of making plausible reasons to justify or explain one's behavior
_____ Suppression	
	g. An individual's incorporation of a characteristic belonging to another person or group
	h. The expression of emotions toward someone or something other than the source of the emotion

6. List several factors associated with the hospital environment that may have an impact on the mental health of a patient who has been hospitalized.

7. Indicate whether each of the following statements is true or false.

a. _____ Reminiscence and life review are ineffective techniques to help the older adult successfully cope with changing life circumstances.

b. _____ Older people experiencing sensory changes may also have behavioral changes that could be mistaken for disorientation.

8. The nurse is caring for an older patient who is exhibiting signs of mental illness. The patient's wife is distraught and asks the nurse how her husband could have seemed fine and now be having these problems. What response by the nurse is most appropriate?
   a. "Mental illness can appear with little or no warning."
   b. "Sadly, he has probably been ill for some time but was able to disguise the symptoms until now."
   c. "Mental health and illness are conditions that can be ever changing based on a person's ability to manage stressors."
   d. "Older adults are prone to mental illness."

9. The nurse is talking with an assigned patient and his spouse. The patient has been admitted to the facility with an acute anxiety disorder. The spouse asks why only one of them has experienced the disorder, even though both have been exposed to the same issues. What response by the nurse is most therapeutic?
   a. "Individual perceptions of stress determine its impact on mental health."
   b. "Different people manage stress differently."
   c. "Mentally ill people are less able to manage life stressors."
   d. "Men are less able to cope with life stressors than women."

Exercise 2

Virtual Hospital Activity

45 minutes

- Sign in to work at Pacific View Regional Hospital for Period of Care 1. (*Note:* If you are already in the virtual hospital from a previous exercise, click on **Leave the Floor** and then **Restart the Program** to get to the sign-in window.)
- From the Patient List, select Carlos Reyes (Room 504).
- Click **Get Report** and read the Clinical Report.
- Click **Go to Nurse's Station**.
- Click **Chart** and then **504** to view Carlos Reyes' chart.
- Click the **History and Physical** and **Nursing Admission** tabs and review the information given.

1. Why is Carlos Reyes being transferred to the Skilled Nursing Unit?

2. List significant factors recorded in Carlos Reyes' past medical history.

3. Describe Carlos Reyes' demeanor during the admission nursing assessment.

4. Identify factors that may influence the amount/degree of anxiety that Carlos Reyes may experience.

5. What does Carlos Reyes' family report concerning his cognitive status?

- Click **Return to Nurses' Station** and then click **504** at the bottom of the screen to enter Carlos Reyes' room.
- Read the **Initial Observations**.
- Click **Take Vital Signs** and review the findings.
- Click and read the **Clinical Alerts**.
- Click **Patient Care** and perform a head-to-toe assessment.

6. List the mental health abnormalities noted during the assessment.

7. What sensory changes associated with aging may further affect Carlos Reyes' ability to respond appropriately to environmental stimuli?

8. What other factors associated with aging may affect Carlos Reyes' mental health?

9. What impact might Carlos Reyes' myocardial infarction have on his mental health?

10. What factors will affect the level of anxiety that Carlos Reyes may experience in response to the stressors being encountered? Select all that apply.

    _____ How the patient views the stressors

    _____ The number of stressors being managed at the same time

    _____ The perception of stress by his health care team

    _____ Past experience with similar situations

    _____ The degree of significance the stressor will have on the future

11. Identify nursing interventions to reduce the stressors associated with Carlos Reyes' hospitalization.

- Click **Patient Care** and then **Nurse-Client Interactions**.
- Select and view the video titled **0740: Family Teaching—Medication**. (*Note:* Check the virtual clock to see whether enough time has elapsed. You can use the fast-forward feature to advance the time by 2-minute intervals if the video is not yet available. Then click again on **Patient Care** and **Nurse-Client Interactions** to refresh the screen.)

12. Describe Carlos Reyes' level of responsiveness in the video.

13. What concerns are being voiced by Carlos Reyes' son?

14. The nurse tells Carlos Reyes' son that his father has been given a medication called

    _____.

- Click **Chart** and then **504** to view Carlos Reyes' chart.
- Click the **Nurse's Notes** tab and review the information given.

15. In addition to the medication prescribed for Carlos Reyes, what other factors may be contributing to his level of responsiveness?

- Click **Return to Room 504**.
- Click the **Drug** icon at the bottom of the screen and review the information for the drug that Carlos Reyes has been given.

16. Which are indications for the administration of this medication? Select all that apply.

    _____ Pain

    _____ Intermittent confusion

    _____ Mild to moderate anxiety

    _____ Severe anxiety

    _____ Hallucinations

    _____ Alcohol withdrawal

17. What side effects may be encountered with the administration of this medication?

18. What safety interventions or precautions should be implemented for the patient taking this drug?

19. What actions have been taken by the nurse in response to the family's concerns and the patient's condition?

Care of the Patient with a Psychiatric Disorder

Reading Assignment: Concepts of Mental Health (Chapter 34)
Care of the Patient with a Psychiatric Disorder (Chapter 35)

Patient: Carlos Reyes, Room 504

Objectives:

1. Identify abnormal findings related to mental health status during a physical assessment.
2. Identify nonverbal cues in the nurse-patient interaction.
3. List nursing interventions to promote and/or develop therapeutic communication.
4. Define the various types of anxiety disorders.
5. List defense mechanisms that may be used by the patient experiencing stress.

Exercise 1

Writing Activity

30 minutes

1. Numerous techniques may be used in psychiatric therapy. Match each therapeutic technique listed below with its correct description.

Therapeutic Technique	**Description**
_____ Behavior therapy	a. The use of toys and puppets to express feelings
_____ Cognitive therapy	b. Used to relieve anxiety by conditioning and retraining responses by repetition
_____ Group therapy	
	c. A long-term process used to bring unconscious feelings to the surface
_____ Play therapy	
_____ Free association	d. Breaking negative thought patterns and developing positive feelings about memories or thoughts
_____ Psychoanalysis	
	e. The joining of patients sharing similar concerns and experiences
	f. Speaking thoughts without censorship

2. What is dementia?

3. What type of dementia is seen most commonly in the United States?

4. Two key elements in the nursing care of patients with dementia are providing a

_____ and using _____ techniques.

5. Which four nursing interventions promote adequate nutrition in a patient with dementia?

6. Identify common problems associated with dementia.

7. What are generalized anxiety disorders?

8. Match each anxiety disorder with its appropriate definition.

Disorder	Definition
_____ Free-floating anxiety	a. An irrational fear in which the person dwells on the object of anxiety
_____ Signal anxiety	
	b. A response to an intense traumatic experience that is beyond the usual range of human experiences
_____ Panic attack	
_____ Phobia	c. A learned response to an event
_____ Obsessive-compulsive disorder	d. Recurrent, intrusive thoughts that produce anxiety and repetitive, ritualistic behaviors
_____ Posttraumatic stress disorder	e. Feelings of dread that cannot be identified
	f. Acute, intense, and overwhelming anxiety accompanied by a degree of personality disorganization and inability to solve problems or think clearly

9. The use of pharmacologic therapies to treat mental health disorders may involve numerous side effects. Match each commonly seen side effect with its correct definition.

Side Effect	Definition
_____ Akathisia	a. Aberrant posturing
_____ Pseudoparkinsonism	b. Involuntary movements
_____ Dystonias	c. An inability to sit still with continuous movements
_____ Dyskinesia	d. Tremor and rigid posture

10. In addition to medications, what "natural" or herbal medications may be used in the treatment of mental health conditions? For what type of condition is each used?

11. What concerns accompany the use of herbal and natural medications?

Exercise 2

Virtual Hospital Activity

30 minutes

- Sign in to work at Pacific View Regional Hospital for Period of Care 2. (*Note:* If you are already in the virtual hospital from a previous exercise, click on **Leave the Floor** and then **Restart the Program** to get to the sign-in window.)
- From the Patient List, select Carlos Reyes (Room 504).
- Click **Get Report** and read the Clinical Report.

1. What are the primary concerns for Carlos Reyes reported from the previous shift?

- Click **Go to Nurses' Station** and then click **504** at the bottom of the screen to enter the patient's room.
- Click **Patient Care** and perform a head-to-toe physical assessment.

2. Several elements associated with Carlos Reyes' mental health indicate impaired mental and cognitive functioning. According to his physical assessment, how would you describe the following?

    a. Orientation:

    b. Level of consciousness:

    c. Concentration:

    d. Memory:

    e. Speech patterns:

    f. Communication:

    g. Mental state:

- Click **Nurse-Client Interactions**.
- Select and view the video titled **1120: The Agitated Patient**. (*Note:* Check the virtual clock to see whether enough time has elapsed. You can use the fast-forward feature to advance the time by 2-minute intervals if the video is not yet available. Then click again on **Patient Care** and **Nurse-Client Interactions** to refresh the screen.)

3. Describe Carlos Reyes' mental status and responses to the nurse's attempt at interaction. Include his nonverbal cues.

4. What interventions can the nurse use to promote and develop therapeutic communication with Carlos Reyes?

- Click **Chart** and then **504** to view Carlos Reyes' chart.
- Click the **Physician's Orders**, **History and Physical**, and **Consultations** tabs and review each section.

5. What is the physician's impression of Carlos Reyes' mental health status as reported in the History and Physical?

6. What consultations have been ordered or completed?

7. Describe the impressions of the discharge planning coordinator.

8. Who is the primary caregiver for Carlos Reyes?

- Click **Return to Room 504**.
- Click **Patient Care** and then **Nurse-Client Interactions**.
- Select and view the videos titled **1140: Assessing for Referrals** and **1145: Intervention—Referral**. (*Note:* Check the virtual clock to see whether enough time has elapsed. You can use the fast-forward feature to advance the time by 2-minute intervals if the video is not yet available. Then click again on **Patient Care** and **Nurse-Client Interactions** to refresh the screen.)

9. How does Carlos Reyes' son feel the hospitalization has affected his father's mental status?

10. Discuss the conflict between Carlos Reyes' children.

11. Listed below are medications and dosages that have been prescribed for Carlos Reyes. Match each medication with its intended use. (*Note:* Answers may be used more than one time.)

Medication	Intended Use
_____ Tacrine 30 mg QID	a. Reduce anxiety
_____ Oxazepam 15 mg TID	b. Increase cognitive functioning
_____ Triazolam 0.125 mg hs	c. Sleep aid
_____ Lorazepam 0.5 mg PO q12h	

12. For each medication that has been prescribed for Carlos Reyes, identify the possible side effects.

   a. Tacrine:

   b. Oxazepam:

   c. Triazolam:

   d. Lorazepam:

13. When administering lorazepam, what precautions should be included in the nurse's plan of care? Select all that apply.

   _____ Administer in the mornings.

   _____ Administer dosage with food.

   _____ Drowsiness usually disappears during continued therapy.

   _____ Monitor vital signs.

   _____ Do not crush medications.

14. Carlos Reyes' physician has prescribed triazolam. When reviewing his history for the use of alternative therapies, what herbal compound would be cause for concern?
   a. St. John's wort
   b. Ginkgo
   c. Kava
   d. Chamomile

LESSON **17**

Assessment of the Patient with Osteomyelitis

Reading Assignment: Care of the Patient with an Integumentary Disorder (Chapter 44)
Care of the Patient with a Musculoskeletal Disorder (Chapter 45)

Patient: Harry George, Room 401

Objectives:

1. Understand the basic functions of the musculoskeletal system.
2. Review the various types of arthritis.
3. Review risk factors for osteomyelitis.
4. Identify the clinical manifestations of osteomyelitis.
5. Discuss treatment options for the patient with osteomyelitis.

Exercise 1

Writing Activity

15 minutes

1. The skeletal system serves five major functions:

    a. The skeleton provides the body _____ that supports internal tissues and organs.

    b. The skeleton forms a _____ that protects many internal organs.

    c. Bones provide _____ for movement.

    d. The bones serve as storage areas for various _____.

    e. _____ (blood cell formation) takes place in the red bone marrow.

2. Match each type of body movement with its correct definition. (*Hint:* See Box 4-2 in your textbook.)

Type of Body Movement	Definition
_____ Abduction	a. Movement of the bone around its longitudinal axis
_____ Adduction	b. Movement that causes the bottom of the foot to be directed downward
_____ Dorsiflexion	c. Movement of certain joints that decreases the angle between two adjoining bones
_____ Extension	
_____ Flexion	d. Movement of the hand and forearm that causes the palm to face downward or backward
_____ Plantar flexion	e. Movement of an extremity toward the axis of the body
_____ Pronation	f. Movement of the hand and forearm that causes the palm to face upward or forward
_____ Rotation	
_____ Supination	g. Movement of certain joints that increases the angle between two adjoining bones
	h. Movement of an extremity away from the midline of the body
	i. Movement that causes the top of the foot to elevate or tilt upward

3. Which muscles are responsible for movement of the lower extremities? Select all that apply.

_____ Gluteus maximus

_____ Soleus

_____ Masseter

_____ Orbicularis oris

_____ Adductor longus

4. List the four most common types of arthritis.

5. The nurse conducts a teaching session for a patient diagnosed with gout. During the discussion, the nurse addresses dietary concerns. Which statements by the patient indicate the need for further instruction? Select all that apply.

_____ "I should avoid hard liquor but can still indulge in beer or wine with my condition."

_____ "Organ meats contain high levels of protein and will help in the management of my condition."

_____ "I will need to avoid yeast-containing products."

_____ "Certain seafood items may be problematic and will need to be avoided."

_____ "I should limit my fluid intake during the flare-ups of my condition."

6. The nurse is reviewing the chart of a patient who is suspected of having rheumatoid arthritis. What findings would be consistent with the condition? Select all that apply.

_____ Complete cell count that indicates a reduced white blood cell count

_____ Bony knobs on the ends of the fingers

_____ Familial history of rheumatoid arthritis

_____ Patient complaints of tenderness of joints

_____ Symmetrical involvement of joints

7. A female patient with a strong family history of osteoarthritis has voiced concerns about the disease. The patient asks what areas of the body are most often affected in her gender. What information can be provided by the nurse?
   a. Osteoarthritis affects the hips of women most often.
   b. Osteoarthritic changes are most often evident in the knees of women.
   c. Osteoarthritis affects the hands of women most often.
   d. Osteoarthritis is seen most often in the lumbosacral region of women most often.

8. Osteomyelitis is an infection of bone and/or bone marrow. What are the most common causes of osteomyelitis?

9. A variety of organisms may cause osteomyelitis. What is the most common causative agent?
   a. *Staphylococcus areus*
   b. *Streptococcus viridans*
   c. *Escherichia coli*
   d. *Neisseria gonorrhoeae*

10. How is osteomyelitis treated?

Exercise 2

Virtual Hospital Activity

45 minutes

- Sign in to work at Pacific View Regional Hospital for Period of Care 1. (*Note:* If you are already in the virtual hospital from a previous exercise, click **Leave the Floor** and then **Restart the Program** to get to the sign-in window.)
- From the Patient List, select Harry George (Room 401).
- Click **Get Report** and read the Clinical Report.
- Click **Go to Nurses' Station**; then click **401** to enter Harry George's room.
- Click **Patient Care** and complete a head-to-toe assessment.

1. When you are assessing Harry George's affected extremity, which factors should you include in the assessment?

2. Harry George was admitted with a diagnosis of osteomyelitis. What findings support this diagnosis?

3. How does the affected extremity appear?

4. How does the assessment of the left (affected) leg differ from that of the right?

5. What other clinical manifestations may accompany a diagnosis of osteomyelitis?

6. How should the affected extremity be positioned?

7. During the head-to-toe assessment, Harry George asks the nurse how long it will take before he "no longer has this nasty infection in his bones." What response by the nurse is most appropriate?
   a. "Once you complete this course of antibiotic therapy, you should have this infection beat."
   b. "You may have this infection for at least another year."
   c. "An infection of the bone is difficult to treat and may be a factor for your entire life."
   d. "It takes at least 6 months to know if and when you will be free of infection."

- Click **Take Vital Signs** and review the information provided.

8. Discuss any findings in Harry George's vital signs that may indicate the presence of infection.

9. What possible complications could Harry George face if osteomyelitis progresses?

- Click **Chart** at the top of the screen.
- Click **401** to view Harry George's chart.
- Click the **Consultations** tab.
- Review the report by the Wound Care Team.

10. What age-related changes will further affect Harry George's ability to achieve wound healing? Select all that apply.

_____ Increases in tissue fluid

_____ Reduced skin elasticity

_____ Reductions in subcutaneous fat

_____ Circulatory changes

11. Which diagnostic tests may be ordered to support a diagnosis of osteomyelitis? Select all that apply.

_____ MRI

_____ PET scan

_____ Bone scan

_____ X-rays

_____ Serum electrolytes

_____ Erythrocyte sedimentation rate

_____ Blood cultures

_____ Cultures of any drainage from open wounds

_____ Complete blood count

- Still in Harry George's chart, click and review the **Laboratory Reports** and the **Diagnostic Reports** sections.

12. What diagnostic tests were ordered for Harry George to support the diagnosis of osteomyelitis?

13. Which lab results support the diagnosis?

14. What findings were reported in the x-ray and bone scan?

- Click the **History and Physical** tab and review this report.

15. Based on your review of Harry George's medical and social history, what risk factors for osteomyelitis does he have?

16. What will be assessed to determine the effectiveness of Harry George's treatment?

Let's jump ahead to a later period of care and check on Harry George's condition.

- Click **Return to Nurses' Station**.
- Click **Leave the Floor**.
- Click **Restart the Program**.
- Sign in to work at Pacific View Regional Hospital for Period of Care 3.
- Select Harry George from the Patient List.
- Click **Go to Nurses' Station**.
- Click **Chart**.
- Click **401**.
- Click the **Physician's Orders** tab and review the orders given.

17. What treatments have been ordered to manage Harry George's osteomyelitis?

18. What consultations have been ordered by the physician to assist in the management of Harry George's care?

- Click **Consultations**.
- Review the Wound Care Team report.

19. What concerns did the Wound Care Team reveal that are seen as detriments to the healing of Harry George's wound? How can these concerns present problems?

20. The nurse is planning to assist Harry George in the selection of foods that are rich in elements to promote wound healing. Which vitamins and mineral(s) should the nurse recognize as vital to his healing? Select all that apply. (*Hint:* See Health Promotion: Healthy Skin in Chapter 2 in your textbook.)

_____   Vitamin A

_____   Vitamin B

_____   Vitamin C

_____   Vitamin D

_____   Calcium

_____   Iron

_____   Magnesium

21. What interventions can the nurse implement to manage the concerns of the Wound Care Team?

- Click **Return to Nurses' Station**.
- Click **MAR** and then click tab **401**.
- Click **Drug Guide**.
- Review the information given.

22. These medications have been prescribed by Harry George's physician. Which are intended to manage his osteomyelitis? Select all that apply.

_____   Gentamicin 20 mg IV

_____   Thiamine 100 mg PO/IM

_____   Glyburide 1.25 mg PO

_____   Cefotaxime 2 g IV

_____   Phenytoin sodium 100 mg

Care of the Patient Experiencing Comorbid Conditions (Musculoskeletal and Endocrine)

Reading Assignment: Care of the Patient with an Endocrine Disorder (Chapter 52)

Patient: Harry George, Room 401

Objectives:

1. Describe the functions of the endocrine system.
2. Describe the use of a sliding insulin scale.
3. Explain how type 1 and type 2 diabetes are similar and how they differ.
4. List disorders of the endocrine system.
5. Describe the tests used to assess for the presence of diabetes.

Exercise 1

Writing Activity

30 minutes

1. Which statements are true regarding the role and/or function of the endocrine and exocrine systems? Select all that apply.

   _____ Endocrine glands are ductless glands.

   _____ Exocrine glands are responsible for reproductive functioning.

   _____ Endocrine glands release their secretions directly into the bloodstream.

   _____ The endocrine system secretes hormones.

   _____ Exocrine glands assist with maintaining homeostasis for the body.

2. The _____ is considered the "master gland" of the endocrine system.

3. _____ is the means by which the endocrine system maintains homeostasis.

4. Match each disorder of the pituitary gland with its correct description.

Disorder of the Pituitary Gland	**Description**
_____ Acromegaly	a. A transient or permanent metabolic disorder of the posterior pituitary in which ADH is deficient
_____ Gigantism	
_____ Dwarfism	b. A disorder in which the pituitary gland releases too much ADH and, in response, the kidneys reabsorb more water
_____ Diabetes insipidus	c. An overproduction of somatotropin in the adult
_____ Syndrome of inappropriate secretion of antidiuretic hormone (SIADH)	d. A condition in which there is a deficiency in growth hormone
	e. A condition that usually results from an oversecretion of growth hormone

5. What is diabetes?

6. For each characteristic listed below, identify whether it is a characteristic of (a) type 1 diabetes mellitus, (b) type 2 diabetes mellitus, or (c) both type 1 and type 2 diabetes mellitus.

Characteristic	**Type of Diabetes**
_____ Usually associated with individuals under age 30	a. Type 1 diabetes mellitus
_____ Underweight	b. Type 2 diabetes mellitus
_____ Overweight	c. Both type 1 and type 2 diabetes mellitus
_____ May be controlled with oral agents	
_____ Incidence of complications	
_____ Gradual onset	

7. A patient recently diagnosed with diabetes mellitus asks the nurse about potential causes. The nurse correctly recognizes that which factors may be considered to have a causative relationship with the disease? Select all that apply.

_____ Obesity

_____ Autoimmune disorder development

_____ Ethnicity

_____ Lifestyle

_____ Caucasian

_____ Genetic factors

8. Match each diagnostic test for diabetes with its function. (*Hint:* See Box 11-2 in your textbook.)

Diagnostic Test	**Function**
_____ Fasting blood glucose	a. Test used to determine the presence of either type 1 or type 2 diabetes mellitus
_____ Postprandial blood glucose	b. The administration of a carbohydrate solution followed by drawing a blood specimen to assess the level of blood glucose hours later
_____ Glycosylated hemoglobin	c. Drawing of a blood sample after a period of fasting, typically 8 hours
_____ C peptide	d. Used to measure the level of glucose that has been incorporated into the body's hemoglobin

9. Match each type of insulin with its onset of action after administration. (*Note:* It is possible that not all options will be used.)

Type of Insulin	Onset of Action After Administration
_____ Lispro	a. 15 to 30 minutes
_____ Regular	b. 30 to 60 minutes
_____ NPH	c. 1 to 2 hours
_____ NPH/regular mix 70/30	d. 4 to 8 hours
_____ Glargine	e. 2 to 4 hours

10. Most available insulin is U/_____.

11. Indicate whether each statement is true or false.

   a. _____ Urine testing is the recommended way of monitoring glucose levels in the IDDM patient.

   b. _____ Lantus should never be mixed with regular insulin.

   c. _____ Patients with diabetes can choose between insulin or oral agents.

12. Insulin should be administered to the _____ tissue.

13. Which is the site with the fastest rate of insulin absorption?
   a. Abdomen
   b. Arms
   c. Thighs
   d. Buttocks

14. Long-term subcutaneous insulin injections can result in a firm lump under the skin, which can impede

   insulin absorption. This is known as _____.

15. The only insulin that can be administered intravenously is _____.

Exercise 2

Virtual Hospital Activity

30 minutes

- Sign in to work at Pacific View Regional Hospital for Period of Care 1. (*Note:* If you are already in the virtual hospital from a previous exercise, click **Leave the Floor** and then **Restart the Program** to get to the sign-in window.)
- From the Patient List, select Harry George (Room 401).
- Click **Get Report** and read the Clinical Report.
- Click **Go to Nurses' Station** and then click **Chart**.

- Click **401** to view Harry George's chart.
- Click the **Emergency Department** tab and review the information given.
- Click the **Laboratory Reports** tab and review the information given.

1. What was Harry George's plasma blood glucose upon his arrival at the emergency department?

2. Harry George's HbA_{1C} is _____.

3. Based on the HbA_{1C} level, what inferences can be made about Harry George's typical blood glucose levels?
   a. Harry George's blood glucose levels are most often between 130 and 150 mg/dL.
   b. Harry George's blood glucose levels are most often between 150 and 175 mg/dL.
   c. Harry George's blood glucose levels are most often between 175 and 200 mg/dL.
   d. Harry George's blood glucose levels most often exceed 200 mg/dL.

4. What is the desired blood glucose level for a patient with diabetes?

5. Which type of diabetes does Harry George have?
   a. Diabetes insipidus
   b. Type 1 diabetes mellitus
   c. Type 2 diabetes mellitus
   d. Prediabetes

6. What medication had Harry George been taking to control his diabetes?

7. Which action best describes the mechanics of the drug you identified in the previous question?
   a. Stimulates the beta cells of the pancreas to release insulin
   b. Works to reduce hepatic glucose production
   c. Works to increase cell receptiveness to the body's natural insulin
   d. Inhibits glucose conversion to glucagon

8. In addition to his daily scheduled medications to control his diabetes, Harry George has a sliding scale. Describe the use of a sliding scale.

9. When caring for Harry George, the nurse notes that his blood glucose level is 134 mg/dL. What actions by the nurse are most appropriate? Select all that apply.

_____ Hold the prescribed dose of oral hypoglycemic medication.

_____ Provide him with a carbohydrate snack.

_____ Notify the health care provider.

_____ Document the findings.

_____ Administer the prescribed oral hypoglycemic medication.

10. During an illness what is the recommended frequency of blood glucose monitoring for the patient?
   a. Hourly
   b. Every 1 to 2 hours
   c. Every 4 hours
   d. Every 8 hours

11. What impact might illness have on Harry George's blood glucose?

12. How does Harry George's diabetes affect his health status? For which additional complications might he be at risk because of his diabetes?

- Click **Return to Nurses' Station**.
- Click **401** at the bottom of the screen to enter Harry George's room.
- Click **Patient Care** and then **Nurse-Client Interactions**.
- Select and view the video titled **0735: Symptom Management**. (*Note:* Check the virtual clock to see whether enough time has elapsed. You can use the fast-forward feature to advance the time by 2-minute intervals if the video is not yet available. Then click again on **Patient Care** and **Nurse-Client Interactions** to refresh the screen.)

13. What nonverbal behaviors are displayed by the patient, indicating a problem that needs to be addressed?

14. During the talk between Harry George and his sitter, what needs and concerns are voiced?

- Click **Chart** and then **401** to view Harry George's chart.
- Click the **Physician's Orders** tab and review the orders.

15. What is the frequency of Harry George's blood glucose assessments?

16. What type of dietary management is being implemented?

17. Which statement concerning Harry George's prescribed diet is correct?
    a. The diet will consist of three full meals per day to prevent snacking.
    b. The fat content should consist of no more than 30% of the caloric intake.
    c. 60% to 70 % of the calories in the diet should be from carbohydrates to ensure energy.
    d. Snacks should be avoided to reduce blood sugar fluctuations.

18. Harry George should be assessed for teaching needed in which areas?

- Click **Return to Room 401**.
- Click **Patient Care** and then **Nurse-Client Interactions**.
- Select and view the video titled **0755: Disease Management**. (*Note:* Check the virtual clock to see whether enough time has elapsed. You can use the fast-forward feature to advance the time by 2-minute intervals if the video is not yet available. Then click again on **Patient Care** and **Nurse-Client Interactions** to refresh the screen.)

19. While talking with his sitter, Harry George continues to voice the need for his own "medication." What technique does the sitter attempt to employ to manage this request?

LESSON **19** ─────────────────────────

Implementing a Plan of Care for the Patient with Osteomyelitis

───

Reading Assignment: Care of the Patient with a Musculoskeletal Disorder (Chapter 4)

Patient: Harry George, Room 401

Objectives:

1. Understand factors that affect pain management.
2. Identify nursing implications for the administration of narcotic analgesics.
3. Set priorities for the care of the patient with osteomyelitis.

x

Exercise 1

Virtual Hospital Activity

60 minutes

- Sign in to work at Pacific View Regional Hospital for Period of Care 2. (*Note:* If you are already in the virtual hospital from a previous exercise, click **Leave the Floor** and then **Restart the Program** to get to the sign-in window.)
- From the Patient List, select Harry George (Room 401).
- Click **Get Report** and read the Clinical Report.
- Click **Go to Nurses' Station** and then **401** to enter Harry George's room.
- Read the **Initial Observations**.
- Click **Patient Care** and complete a head-to-toe assessment.

1. What are the two primary priorities for Harry George's care at this time?

2. What elements of the assessment or the clinical report did you use to make this decision?

3. How has pain interfered with Harry George's recovery?

4. Is Harry George's pain a new problem or one that has been ongoing? Give a rationale for your response.

5. What nonpharmacologic interventions can be used to attempt to increase Harry George's level of comfort?

- Click **Patient Care** and then **Nurse-Client Interactions**.
- Select and view the video titled **1120: Wound Management**. (*Note:* Check the virtual clock to see whether enough time has elapsed. You can use the fast-forward feature to advance the time by 2-minute intervals if the video is not yet available. Then click again on **Patient Care** and **Nurse-Client Interactions** to refresh the screen.)

6. What behaviors demonstrated by Harry George further support his report of pain and his level of anxiety?

- Now select and view the video titled **1125: Injury Prevention**. (*Note:* Check the virtual clock to see whether enough time has elapsed. You can use the fast-forward feature to advance the time by 2-minute intervals if the video is not yet available. Then click again on **Patient Care** and **Nurse-Client Interactions** to refresh the screen.)

7. During the interaction with his sitter, Harry George continues to appear nervous. His movements reflect jitteriness, and his extremities are trembling. To what can these behaviors be attributed?

- Click **MAR** and then tab **401** to review Harry George's MAR.

8. The physician has prescribed chlordiazepoxide hydrochloride. Other than anxiety, what is an indication for the use of this medication?

9. Which nursing implications are indicated with the administration of chlordiazepoxide hydrochloride? Select all that apply.

_____ Assess vital signs before administration.

_____ Increase ambulation immediately after administration.

_____ Administer cautiously in patients with liver impairments.

_____ Institute safety precautions in regard to ambulation.

_____ This medication may be used in patients who have recently ingested alcohol.

10. In addition to the chlordiazepoxide, what alternative(s) has the physician ordered to reduce Harry George's anxiety?

11. What factors will determine which of the medications should be given?

12. What medication has been ordered to manage Harry George's pain?

13. Does Harry George have any allergies that prevent him from being medicated with the drug prescribed? (*Hint:* Check his armband.)

14. Harry George's last dose of medication for pain was given at _____.

- Click **Return to Room 401**. Then click the **Drug** icon.
- Review the information provided for the medication you identified in question 12.

15. What elements of Harry George's medical/social history should be taken into consideration when administering this drug?

16. The registered nurse has administered this medication by the intravenous route. For which signs of an overdose should the nurse monitor?

17. Are there any special considerations to address when administering this drug in conjunction with the other medications currently in use?

18. Identify any safety measures that should be observed after administration of this medication.

19. Is it time for Harry George to be medicated again for pain?

- Click **Return to Room 401**. Then click **Take Vital Signs**.

20. What are Harry George's vital signs? (*Note:* Exact findings will vary depending on the virtual time at which they are taken.)

    BP:

    SpO$_2$:

    T:

    HR:

    RR:

    Pain:

21. What impact has Harry George's pain had on his vital signs?

22. Are Harry George's vital signs within acceptable limits to administer the drug that has been ordered to manage his pain?

23. If Harry George is unable to take his prescribed medications, what action(s) would be appropriate?

Postoperative Assessment

Reading Assignment: Care of the Surgical Patient (Chapter 43)
Care of the Patient with a Musculoskeletal Disorder (Chapter 45)

Patient: Clarence Hughes, Room 404

Objectives:

1. Define degenerative joint disease.
2. Identify the clinical signs and symptoms of degenerative joint disease.
3. Recognize priorities in nursing diagnoses for the patient who has undergone joint replacement surgery.

Exercise 1

Writing Activity

15 minutes

1. _____ and _____ are two other names for degenerative joint disease.

2. Which populations are at increased risk for developing degenerative joint disease? Select all that apply.

   _____ Small-framed patients

   _____ Obese patients

   _____ Older patients

   _____ Patients employed in occupations with activities that place joints in stressful positions

   _____ Women of childbearing age

   _____ Patients with diabetes

3. The nurse is reviewing the medical record of a patient suspected of having degenerative joint disease. Which findings are considered consistent with degenerative joint disease? Select all that apply.

   _____ Symmetrical joint discomfort

   _____ Family history of degenerative joint disease

   _____ Changes in joint function noted in hands and hips

   _____ Localized pain and stiffness in affected joints

   _____ Warmth over affected joints

4. What are some management techniques for degenerative joint disease?

5. What is arthroscopy?

6. The nurse is reviewing the laboratory results for the patient with suspected degenerative joint disorder. What results support this potential diagnosis? Select all that apply.

_____ Erythrocyte sedimentation rate 12 mm/hr

_____ Rheumatoid factor (RF) 65 units/mL

_____ Uric acid 10.1 mg/dL

_____ Calcium 10 mg/dL

_____ Alkaline phosphatase 43 units/mL

Exercise 2

Virtual Hospital Activity

45 minutes

- Sign in to work at Pacific View Regional Hospital for Period of Care 1. (*Note:* If you are already in the virtual hospital from a previous exercise, click **Leave the Floor** and then **Restart the Program** to get to the sign-in window.)
- From the Patient List, select Clarence Hughes (Room 404).
- Click **Get Report** and read the Clinical Report.
- Click **Go to Nurses' Station** and then **404** to enter Clarence Hughes' room.
- Read the **Initial Observations**.
- Click **Chart** and then **404** to view Clarence Hughes' chart.
- Click the **History and Physical** tab and review the information given.

1. What signs and symptoms of degenerative joint disease has Clarence Hughes experienced?

2. What other methods of disease management did Clarence Hughes try before he had surgery?

- Click **Return to Room 404**.
- Click **Clinical Alerts** and read the information given.
- Now click **Patient Care** and complete a head-to-toe assessment.

3. _____ Findings from Clarence Hughes' physical assessment warrant physician notification. (True/False)

4. What are the two most important priorities for care at this time?

5. Which are the two priority nursing diagnoses for this patient?

6. Why are these issues most important to the successful management of Clarence Hughes' care?

7. Are there any abnormal findings in the abdominal assessment?

- Click **MAR** and then tab **404** to review Clarence Hughes' record.

8. What medication options are available to manage Clarence Hughes' pain?

- Click **Return to Room 404**.
- Click the **Drug** icon and review the pain medication(s) prescribed for Clarence Hughes.

9. Does Clarence Hughes have any contraindications for the pain medication(s) you identified in question 8?

10. What side effects can be anticipated with administration of the medication(s)?

11. Discuss any safety precautions that may need to be instituted with use of the medication(s).

12. Discuss any special monitoring that will be needed with the administration of the medication(s).

13. What regularly scheduled medication has been ordered to reduce the patient's constipation? What is the mechanism of action for this medication?

14. What prn medications have been ordered to reduce constipation? How do these medications work?

- Click **Return to Room 404**.
- Click **Chart** and then **404** to view Clarence Hughes' chart.
- Click the **Physician's Notes** tab.

15. What are the physician's plans concerning Clarence Hughes' discharge?

- Click the **Consultations** tab.

16. What consultations have been ordered for Clarence Hughes? What is the purpose of these consultations?

- Click the **Patient Education** tab.

17. What are Clarence Hughes' educational needs?

18. List five benefits of early postoperative ambulation.

- Click the **Physician's Orders** tab.

19. When does the surgeon request that physical therapy begin?
    a. Physical therapy will begin the day of surgery.
    b. Physical therapy will begin the day after surgery.
    c. Physical therapy will begin on a limited basis 3 to 5 days after surgery.
    d. Physical therapy will be prescribed to start at the time of discharge.

20. What are the physician orders and expectations for use of the continuous passive motion (CPM) machine?

21. Clarence Hughes' physician has ordered use of a CPM machine. Which term best describes the action of this device?
    a. Passive flexion
    b. Active flexion
    c. Passive extension
    d. Active extension

Postoperative Complications

Reading Assignment: Care of the Surgical Patient (Chapter 43)
Care of the Patient with a Respiratory Disorder (Chapter 50)

Patient: Clarence Hughes, Room 404

Objectives:

1. Identify potential postoperative complications.
2. Recognize clinical manifestations associated with the development of postoperative complications.
3. Review the management/treatment of a postoperative complication involving the respiratory system.

Exercise 1

Writing Activity

15 minutes

1. List several potential postoperative complications.

2. The collapse of lung tissue, which results in the lack of adequate exchange of oxygen and carbon

   dioxide, is known as _____.

3. What is a pulmonary embolism?

4. When assessing the patient for a pulmonary embolism, which manifestation(s) can be anticipated? Select all that apply.

   _____ Dull and achy pain

   _____ Pain often described as sharp

   _____ Pain that radiates to the back and neck

   _____ Nonradiating pain

   _____ Dyspnea

   _____ Reduced respiratory rate

   _____ Increased respiratory rate

   _____ Increased pain with inspiration

5. During the initial period after the onset and subsequent diagnosis of a pulmonary embolism, which treatment(s) can be anticipated? Select all that apply.

_____ Oxygen

_____ Oral anticoagulants

_____ Intramuscular antibiotics

_____ Intravenous anticoagulants

_____ Hydration

6. How is a pulmonary embolism managed?

7. What is the prognosis for a patient who develops a pulmonary embolism?

8. Which diagnostic test provides the best visualization of pulmonary vessels to detect a pulmonary embolism?
   a. Chest radiography
   b. Ventilation perfusion scan
   c. CT scan
   d. Pulmonary angiography

Exercise 2

Virtual Hospital Activity

30 minutes

- Sign in to work at Pacific View Regional Hospital for Period of Care 2. (*Note:* If you are already in the virtual hospital from a previous exercise, click **Leave the Floor** and then **Restart the Program** to get to the sign-in window.)
- From the Patient List, select Clarence Hughes (Room 404).
- Click **Get Report** and read the Clinical Report.

1. Are there any abnormal observations in the report?

2. Review the vital signs recorded in the change-of-shift report. Are they normal?

- Click **Go to Nurses' Station**.
- Click **404** at the bottom of the screen to enter the patient's room.
- Read the **Initial Observations**.
- Click **Clinical Alerts** and read the information provided.

3. Which clinical findings indicate a problem?

- Click **Take Vital Signs**.

4. What are Clarence Hughes' current vital signs?

   BP:

   T:

   HR:

   RR:

5. Are any of the above results abnormal? If so, which?

6. What is Clarence Hughes' current oxygen saturation? Is this a normal value? If not, how should it be managed?

- Click **Patient Care** and then **Nurse-Client Interactions**.
- Select and view the video titled **1115: Interventions—Airway**. (*Note:* Check the virtual clock to see whether enough time has elapsed. You can use the fast-forward feature to advance the time by 2-minute intervals if the video is not yet available. Then click again on **Patient Care** and **Nurse-Client Interactions** to refresh the screen.)

7. What behavioral cues being demonstrated by Clarence Hughes indicate a potential health concern?

8. Several nursing interventions are indicated after the onset of Clarence Hughes' breathing problems. Match the columns below to show the order in which these interventions need to be completed.

Nursing Intervention	**Priority Level**
_____ Notify the physician.	a. First
_____ Maintain the airway.	b. Second
_____ Complete a focused assessment.	c. Third
_____ Document care provided.	d. Fourth
_____ Provide education to the family concerning what is taking place.	e. Fifth

- Click **Physical Assessment** and complete a head-to-toe assessment.

9. Are there any significant findings identified in the integumentary assessment?

10. Are there any significant findings identified in the respiratory assessment?

11. Clarence Hughes should be placed in _____ position to facilitate air exchange.

- Click **Chart** and then **404** to view Clarence Hughes' chart.
- Click the **Physician's Orders** tab and review the orders listed for 1120 on Wednesday.

12. What tests and interventions has the physician ordered?

13. The degree of anxiety is often directly tied to the amount of _____ hunger being experienced by the patient.

• Click **Return to Room 404**.
• Click **Patient Care** and then **Nurse-Client Interactions**.
• Select and view the video titled **1135: Change in Patient Condition**. (*Note:* Check the virtual clock to see whether enough time has elapsed. You can use the fast-forward feature to advance the time by 2-minute intervals if the video is not yet available. Then click again on **Patient Care** and **Nurse-Client Interactions** to refresh the screen.)

14. Now that the initial crisis has passed, what are the nurse's priorities concerning the family members?

Exercise 3

Virtual Hospital Activity

15 minutes

• Sign in to work at Pacific View Regional Hospital for Period of Care 3. (*Note:* If you are already in the virtual hospital from the previous exercise, click **Leave the Floor** and then **Restart the Program** to get to the sign-in window.)
• From the Patient List, select Clarence Hughes (Room 404).
• Click **Get Report** and read the report.

1. Give the results for each of the tests listed below.

   a. Arterial blood gas:

   b. Chest x-ray:

   c. Ventilation perfusion scan:

   d. Doppler study:

• Click **Go to Nurses' Station**.
• Click **404** at the bottom of the screen to enter Clarence Hughes' room.
• Read the **Initial Observations**.
• Click and review the **Clinical Alerts**.

2. What changes are noted in the patient's demeanor and clinical manifestations?

- Click **Take Vital Signs** and review the results.

3. What is the significance of the increasing SpO_2 level?

- Click **Chart** and then **404** to review Clarence Hughes' chart.
- Click the **Physician's Orders** tab and review the information given.

4. What medication has been ordered to manage Clarence Hughes' condition? Describe the administration of this medication.

5. What is the method of action and the purpose for the administration of this medication?

6. What is the classification of this medication?

7. During therapy with the medication identified in question 4, which laboratory test is most important to monitor?
   a. PTT
   b. Hgb
   c. Hct
   d. WBC
   e. ESR

8. Once the intravenous anticoagulant therapy has been tapered off, Clarence Hughes can anticipate continuing on oral therapy for a period of:
   a. 3 months.
   b. 6 months.
   c. 9 months.
   d. 1 year.
   e. 18 months.

LESSON **22**

Care of the Patient with Pneumonia

Reading Assignment: Care of the Patient with a Respiratory Disorder (Chapter 50)

Patient: Patricia Newman, Room 406

Objectives:

1. Define pneumonia.
2. Identify the potential causes of pneumonia.
3. Identify the populations at risk for pneumonia.
4. Discuss nursing care for the patient with pneumonia.

Exercise 1

Writing Activity

30 minutes

1. What is pneumonia?

2. Infants and _____ are most susceptible to pneumonia.

3. What factors may increase susceptibility to pneumonia?

4. Which factors may contribute to the development of pneumonia? Select all that apply.

_____ Overuse of steroid medications

_____ Infection

_____ Hyperventilation

_____ Inadequate ventilation

_____ Aspiration

_____ Poor nutritional habits

5. Match the columns below to show the correct order of pathologic occurrences associated with the development of pneumonia.

Disease Process	**Order of Occurrence**
_____ The respiratory tract develops inflammation and localized edema.	a. First
	b. Second
_____ The exchange of oxygen and carbon dioxide becomes increasingly reduced.	c. Third
_____ Secretions begin to accumulate and are not able to be moved by the cilia in the lungs.	d. Fourth
_____ Retained secretions become infected.	

6. When caring for a patient diagnosed with pneumonia, which nursing interventions are appropriate? Select all that apply.

_____ Keep patient on complete bedrest.

_____ Encourage deep breathing and coughing activities.

_____ Initiate exercise training.

_____ Provide patient education aimed at reducing the spread of infection.

_____ Restrict protein intake.

_____ Monitor vital signs and pulmonary status.

_____ Provide information concerning the prescribed medication therapy.

_____ Encourage fluid intake if not contraindicated by patient's coexisting conditions.

7. What is the typical prognosis for a patient with pneumonia?

8. When assisting the patient with pneumonia to plan meals, which dietary recommendation should be implemented?
   a. Three large balanced meals each day will be best to provide the needed nutrients.
   b. The diet should include at least 3000 calories per day.
   c. Increased amounts of protein and sodium are indicated.
   d. The diet should consist of at least 1500 calories each day.

9. What is the purpose of the above dietary intervention?

10. The patient with pneumonia should consume at least _____ of fluid per day unless contra-indicated by other medical conditions.

Exercise 2

Virtual Hospital Activity

30 minutes

- Sign in to work at Pacific View Regional Hospital for Period of Care 1. (*Note:* If you are already in the virtual hospital from a previous exercise, click **Leave the Floor** and then **Restart the Program** to get to the sign-in window.)
- From the Patient List, select Patricia Newman (Room 406).
- Click **Get Report** and read the Clinical Report.
- Click **Go to Nurses' Station**.
- Click **Chart** and then **406** to view Patricia Newman's chart.
- Click the **Emergency Department** tab and review the information given.

1. What were the findings of the Initial Assessment in the emergency department?

2. Discuss any abnormal findings in her respiratory system assessment.

3. Find the vital sign results on the ED record and discuss the significance of these findings.

4. What are the primary and secondary admitting diagnoses?

5. Listed below are laboratory tests ordered for Patricia Newman while in the emergency department. Match each laboratory test with its reason for being ordered.

Laboratory Test	**Reason It Was Ordered**
_____ Sputum gram stain	a. To provide information about the potential presence of infection and the body's response
_____ Arterial blood gases	b. To identify specific pathogens in a specimen
_____ Complete blood count	c. To identify the specific pathogens and determine which medications therapies will be most effective
_____ Culture and sensitivity	
_____ Erythrocyte sedimentation rate	d. To identify the presence and degree of inflammation in the body
	e. To definitely evaluate the oxygen levels in the body

6. Patricia Newman's physician has ordered a chest x-ray. What is the rationale for ordering this test?

- Click **Return to Nurses' Station**.
- Click **406** at the bottom of the screen and review the **Initial Observations**.

7. Discuss the significance of the oxygen saturation and the patient's removal of the nasal cannula.

- Click **Return to Room 406**.
- Click **Take Vital Signs** and review the results provided.

8. What are the patient's current vital signs, including oxygen saturation and pain level?

   BP:

   SpO$_2$:

   T:

   HR:

   RR:

   Pain:

9. Review Patricia Newman's vital signs listed in the previous question. What is the significance of these findings?

- Click **Patient Care** and complete a head-to-toe assessment.

10. What assessment findings support the admitting diagnosis of pneumonia?

- Click **MAR** and then tab **406** to review the medications ordered for Patricia Newman.

11. The following drugs have been ordered to manage Patricia Newman's pneumonia. Match each drug with its correct classification.

Drug	Classification
_____ Acetaminophen	a. Antipyretic
_____ Cefotan	b. Antiinflammatory
_____ Ipratropium	c. Antibiotic
	d. Bronchodilator
	e. Corticosteroid

- Click **Return to Room 406**.
- Click **Chart** and then **406** to view Patricia Newman's chart.
- Click the **Laboratory Reports** tab and review the information given.

12. Patricia Newman had arterial blood gases drawn on Wednesday. Review her results below. Which are within normal limits? Select all that apply.

_____ pH: 7.33

_____ PaO_2: 70 mm Hg

_____ $PaCO_2$: 47 mm Hg

13. Review Patricia Newman's arterial gas pH level of 7.33. What is this level most reflective of?
    a. Acidity
    b. Alkalinity

14. With consideration to the pH, PO_2, and PCO_2 levels, which interpretation of the arterial blood gases is most likely?
    a. Metabolic acidosis
    b. Metabolic alkalosis
    c. Respiratory acidosis
    d. Respiratory alkalosis

15. Discuss the significance of the culture and sensitivity test results.

16. Review and discuss the findings of the complete blood count test.

- Click the **Diagnostic Reports** tab and review the report.

17. Review the chest x-ray. What findings are consistent with the diagnosis of pneumonia?

18. Which clinical manifestations will reflect positive impact of treatments?

19. _____ Patricia Newman should take the pneumococcal vaccine. (True/False)

Care of the Patient Experiencing Comorbid Conditions (Musculoskeletal and Respiratory)

Reading Assignment: Care of the Patient with a Musculoskeletal Disorder (Chapter 45)
Care of the Patient with a Cardiovascular or a Peripheral Vascular Disorder (Chapter 49)
Care of the Patient with a Respiratory Disorder (Chapter 50)

Patient: Patricia Newman, Room 406

Objectives:

1. Identify significant findings in a patient's medical history.
2. Identify significant findings in a patient's social history.
3. Discuss the pathophysiology, risk factors, and management of hypertension.
4. Discuss the pathophysiology, risk factors, and management of osteoporosis.
5. Discuss the pathophysiology, risk factors, and management of emphysema.
6. Identify important issues in caring for the patient with comorbid conditions.

Exercise 1

Writing Activity

30 minutes

1. Which definition most closely describes hypertension?
   a. Sustained diastolic blood pressure of greater than 80 mm Hg
   b. Sustained systolic blood pressure of greater than 140 mm Hg
   c. Sustained systolic blood pressure of greater than 90 mm Hg
   d. Sustained blood pressure reading of 120/80 mm Hg

2. Which risk factors are associated with hypertension? Select all that apply.

   _____ Obesity

   _____ Genetic factors

   _____ Sedentary lifestyle

   _____ Marijuana use

   _____ Asthma

   _____ Increased sodium intake

   _____ Excessive alcohol ingestion

3. List three medical management options for the treatment of hypertension.

4. What is emphysema?

5. Which are risk factors associated with emphysema? Select all that apply.

_____ Family history

_____ History of diabetes

_____ Cigarette use

_____ Environmental exposure to dust

_____ Having worked as a grain bin operator

6. Which are clinical manifestations associated with emphysema? Select all that apply.

_____ Dyspnea with exertion

_____ Hypertension

_____ Tachypnea

_____ Bradypnea

_____ Tachycardia

_____ Bradycardia

_____ Pursed-lip breathing

_____ Weight gain

_____ Barrel-chested appearance

_____ Clubbing of fingers

7. What is the usual prognosis for a patient diagnosed with emphysema?

8. Osteoporosis is a disease characterized by the reduction in _____.

9. Which populations are at high risk for the development of osteoporosis? Select all that apply.

_____ Women

_____ Large-framed individuals

_____ Smokers

_____ People with sedentary lifestyles

_____ People taking supplements to increase calcium intake

_____ Users of steroids

_____ Immobilized individuals

_____ Postmenopausal women

_____ African Americans

10. What areas of the body are most affected by osteoporosis?

11. A nurse is planning care for a patient suspected of having osteoporosis. Which tests may be used to confirm the diagnosis? Select all that apply.

_____ Chest x-ray

_____ CBC

_____ Bone mineral density test

_____ Thyroid function tests

_____ Liver function test

_____ EMG

12. List several clinical manifestations associated with osteoporosis.

13. When planning the care of a patient diagnosed with osteoporosis, the nurse knows that which interventions may be included? Select all that apply.

_____   Exercise

_____   Restricted levels of activity

_____   Increased calcium intake/supplements

_____   Estrogen therapy

_____   Reduced animal protein intake

14. When planning a diet high in calcium, which foods should be included?
   a. Yellow vegetables
   b. Tomatoes
   c. Dates and legumes
   d. Green leafy vegetables

Exercise 2

Virtual Hospital Activity

45 minutes

- Sign in to work at Pacific View Regional Hospital for Period of Care 3. (*Note:* If you are already in the virtual hospital from a previous exercise, click **Leave the Floor** and then **Restart the Program** to get to the sign-in window.)
- From the Patient List, select Patricia Newman (Room 406).
- Click **Go to Nurses' Station**.
- Click **Chart** and then click **406**.
- Click the **History and Physical** tab and review the information provided.

   1. What significant medical issues are in Patricia Newman's medical history?

   2. The coexistence of osteoporosis, emphysema, and hypertension presents what unique problems for Patricia Newman?

3. Does the patient have any surgeries in her medical history?

4. Describe Patricia Newman's social history.

- Still in Patricia Newman's chart, click the **Nursing Admission** tab and review the information given.
- Click the **Laboratory Reports** tab and review the test results.

5. What factors in Patricia Newman's history are related to a diagnosis of emphysema?

6. How is her recurring history of pneumonia related to her emphysema?

7. Review Patricia Newman's medical history. Which findings are associated with her diagnosis of osteoporosis? Select all that apply.

_____ Age

_____ Gender

_____ Sedentary lifestyle

_____ Tobacco use

_____ Underweight status

8. Patricia Newman has which type of pneumonia?
   a. Bacterial pneumonia
   b. Viral pneumonia
   c. Aspiration pneumonia

- Click **Return to Nurses' Station**.
- Click **406** at the bottom of the screen to go to Patricia Newman's room.
- Click **Take Vital Signs** and review the results.
- Next, click **Patient Care** and perform a focused physical assessment.

9. What vital signs and/or assessment findings are consistent with a diagnosis of pneumonia?

- Now click **MAR**.
- Click tab **406** to view the medications ordered for Patricia Newman.

10. What medications have been prescribed to manage Patricia Newman's hypertension?

11. Describe the mode of action for each of the medications that you identified in question 10.

12. When you are planning care for the patient being treated with the above medications, which laboratory test must be monitored?
    a. Serum sodium levels
    b. Serum potassium levels
    c. Erythrocyte sedimentation rate
    d. Complete blood count results

13. What medications have been ordered to manage Patricia Newman's emphysema?

14. What medication has been prescribed to manage Patricia Newman's osteoporosis?

15. After reviewing Patricia Newman's medical history, the nurse recognizes that which is the appropriate amount of calcium to be included in her daily diet?
    a. 750 mg
    b. 1000 mg
    c. 1250 mg
    d. 1500 mg

16. Which nursing implications are indicated when administering the medication ordered to manage osteoporosis? Select all that apply.

    _____ Administer medication 15 to 30 minutes before eating.

    _____ Administer medication with coffee to prevent constipation.

    _____ Administer medication 30 to 60 minutes after eating.

    _____ Monitor blood pressure.

    _____ Administer medication with foods high in fiber.

Prioritizing Care for the Patient with a Pulmonary Disorder

Reading Assignment: Care of the Patient with a Respiratory Disorder (Chapter 50)

Patient: Patricia Newman, Room 406

Objectives:

1. Review the diagnostic tests performed on the patient with emphysema.
2. Identify the primary patient education goals for the patient experiencing a pulmonary disorder.
3. Discuss the appropriate service consultations for a patient experiencing a pulmonary disorder.
4. Determine the impact of personal/social factors in the patient's recovery period.
5. Develop priorities for the patient during hospitalization and in preparation for discharge.

Exercise 1

Writing Activity

30 minutes

1. Which are characteristics associated with emphysema? Select all that apply.

_____ The most common cause of emphysema is cigarette smoking.

_____ Emphysema symptoms typically begin to manifest while the patient is in the mid- to late 30s.

_____ The disorder is characterized by changes in the alveolar walls and capillaries.

_____ Disability often results in patients diagnosed with emphysema between ages 50 and 60 years.

_____ Heredity may play a role in the development of emphysema.

2. When diagnostic tests are ordered to confirm the presence of emphysema, which tests may be anticipated? Select all that apply.

_____ Thoracentesis

_____ Arterial blood gases

_____ Complete blood cell count

_____ Chest x-ray

_____ Bronchoscopy

_____ Pulse oximetry

3. When caring for a patient diagnosed with emphysema, the nurse should anticipate which result for a pulmonary function test?
   a. Reduced residual volume
   b. Reduced airway resistance
   c. Increased ventilatory response
   d. Increased residual volume

4. The complete blood cell count will reflect which result(s) in a patient diagnosed with emphysema?
   a. Reduced erythrocyte count
   b. Elevated erythrocyte count
   c. Elevated erythrocyte count and reduced hemoglobin
   d. Reduced erythrocyte count and elevated hemoglobin

5. In the patient who is experiencing emphysema, which result best reflects the anticipated pulmonary function tests?
   a. Increased PaO_2
   b. Decreased total lung capacity
   c. Reduced residual volume
   d. Increased total lung capacity

6. Describe the disease process associated with emphysema.

7. Indicate whether each statement is true or false.

    a. _____   An inherited form of emphysema is due to an oversecretion of a liver protein known as ATT.

    b. _____   Hypercapnia does not develop until the later stages of emphysema.

8. Discuss the use of exercise in the care and management of the patient diagnosed with emphysema.

9. _____ is an abnormal cardiac condition characterized by hypertrophy of the right ventricle of the heart due to hypertension of the pulmonary circulation.

10. What are the management options for the patient with emphysema?

Exercise 2

Virtual Hospital Activity

30 minutes

- Sign in to work at Pacific View Regional Hospital for Period of Care 3. (*Note:* If you are already in the virtual hospital from a previous exercise, click **Leave the Floor** and then **Restart the Program** to get to the sign-in window.)
- From the Patient List, select Patricia Newman (Room 406).
- Click **Get Report** and read the Clinical Report.
- Click **Go to Nurses' Station**.
- Click **406** at the bottom of the screen. Read the **Initial Observations**.
- Click **Patient Care** and then **Nurse-Client Interactions**.
- Select and view the video titled **1500: Discharge Planning**. (*Note:* Check the virtual clock to see whether enough time has elapsed. You can use the fast-forward feature to advance the time by 2-minute intervals if the video is not yet available. Then click again on **Patient Care** and **Nurse-Client Interactions** to refresh the screen.)

1. Discuss Patricia Newman's demeanor during the video interaction.

2. What appear to be the patient's biggest concerns during this interaction?

- Click **Physical Assessment** and complete a head-to-toe assessment.

3. What evidence suggests that Patricia Newman's condition is improving?

4. Are there any assessment findings that could potentially have a negative implication for Patricia Newman's discharge to home? If so, explain.

5. When preparing to discharge Patricia Newman, the nurse will need to review the patient's understanding of the correct use of the metered inhaler. Which observation would indicate the need for additional teaching?
   a. Patricia Newman rinses her mouth out with water immediately after inhalation.
   b. Patricia Newman waits 1 minute between inhaling her first and her second dose.
   c. Patricia Newman shakes the medicine container before use.
   d. Patricia Newman holds her breath as long as she can after administering the medication.

6. As you follow Patricia Newman's plan of care, which are priorities at this time? Select all that apply.

   _____ Dietary counseling

   _____ Preparation for discharge

   _____ Referrals for smoking cessation programs

   _____ Requesting a consultation with physical therapy

   _____ Requesting a consultation with social services

7. Of the nursing diagnoses most likely to be included in the plan of care, which are the top three priority nursing diagnoses?

- Click **Chart** and then **406** to view Patricia Newman's chart.
- Click the **Nursing Admission** tab and review the information given.

8. Identify Patricia Newman's social concerns.

9. Which statement accurately reflects an aspect of Patricia Newman's needs?
    a. She has numerous friends and family members available to provide assistance.
    b. She appears self-sufficient and needs little outside help.
    c. She is somewhat socially isolated.
    d. Her significant other will be available as needed for assistance after discharge.

10. Discuss the implications of these social concerns on the nurse's plan of care for Patricia Newman.

• Click the **Consultations** tab and review the dietary consultation.

11. Which dietary recommendations should be reinforced with Patricia Newman's patient teaching? Select all that apply.

    _____ Avoid resting before eating.

    _____ Recommended oral fluid intake should be 1 to 2 L/day.

    _____ 5 to 6 meals per day are recommended.

    _____ Meals should be high in calories.

    _____ Meals should be low in fiber.

    _____ Moderate protein is recommended.

• Click the **Patient Education** tab and review the information given.

12. As Patricia Newman prepares to go home, which are educational goals for her discharge? Select all that apply.

    _____ Correct use of MDI and peak flow meter

    _____ Understanding the rationale for and performance of pursed-lip breathing and effective cough technique

    _____ The need to be sedentary to avoid further complications

    _____ Understanding of and compliance with her prescribed medication therapy

    _____ Compliance with progressive activity/exercise goals

13. Considering Patricia Newman's social and financial history, which goals may be a challenge for her to meet?

14. When discussing immunization recommendations with Patricia Newman, what information should be included?
    a. The pneumonia vaccine is recommended every 2 years.
    b. The pneumonia vaccine cannot be taken during the same season as the influenza vaccine.
    c. The influenza vaccine is recommended each year.
    d. The influenza vaccine and the pneumonia vaccine are recommended each year.

- Click the **Physician's Orders** tab.

15. What consultations have been ordered for Patricia Newman during this hospitalization?

LESSON **25**

Care of the Patient Experiencing Exacerbation of an Asthmatic Condition

Reading Assignment: Care of the Patient with a Respiratory Disorder (Chapter 50)

Patient: Jacquline Catanazaro, Room 402

Objectives:

1. Define asthma.
2. Identify factors that contribute to an asthmatic episode.
3. Report assessment findings consistent with an exacerbation of asthma.
4. Discuss the impact of emotional distress on the respiratory system.

Exercise 1

Writing Activity

15 minutes

1. What is asthma?

2. Which statement concerning the mechanisms of asthma is true?
   a. Air tubes narrow as a result of swollen tissues and excessive mucus production.
   b. Edema of the respiratory mucosa and excessive mucus production occur, thus obstructing airways.
   c. The walls of the alveoli are torn and cannot be repaired.
   d. The bronchioles are scarred and unable to expand.

3. List the clinical manifestations of mild asthma.

4. List the signs and symptoms associated with an acute asthmatic attack.

5. Which events can trigger an asthmatic episode? Select all that apply.

   _____ Hormone levels

   _____ Mental and physical fatigue

   _____ Emotional factors

   _____ Environmental exposures

   _____ Electrolyte imbalances

6. When an asthmatic condition is suspected, which diagnostic tests will confirm a diagnosis? Select all that apply.

   _____ Platelet count

   _____ Serum electrolyte levels

   _____ Arterial blood gas

   _____ Pulmonary function tests

   _____ Sputum cultures

7. A _____ should be obtained to rule out a secondary infection.

8. When a patient is experiencing an asthma attack, a complete blood cell count will show an elevation in which blood cell type?
   a. Eosinophils
   b. Platelets
   c. Red blood cells
   d. Monocytes

9. A patient experiencing a severe, life-threatening exacerbation of asthma will likely have which peak flow meter reading?
   a. 100%
   b. 45%
   c. 55%
   d. 85%

Exercise 2

Virtual Hospital Activity

45 minutes

- Sign in to work at Pacific View Regional Hospital for Period of Care 1. (*Note:* If you are already in the virtual hospital from a previous exercise, click **Leave the Floor** and then **Restart the Program** to get to the sign-in window.)
- From the Patient List, select Jacquline Catanazaro (Room 402).
- Click **Get Report** and read the Clinical Report.
- Click **Go to Nurses' Station**.
- Click **Chart** and then **402** to view Jacquline Catanazaro's chart.
- Click the **Emergency Department** tab and review the information given.

1. Review the admitting vital signs. What is the significance of the findings?

2. What is the primary admitting diagnosis?

- Click **Return to Nurses' Station** and then **402** at the bottom of the screen.
- Read the **Initial Observations**.
- Click **Take Vital Signs** and review the results.
- Click **Clinical Alerts** and read the report.

3. Jacquline Catanazaro is demonstrating extreme agitation. What is the impact of this on her health status?

4. When preparing to perform a pulse oximeter reading on Jacquline Catanazaro, which sites would be appropriate for this test? Select all that apply.

_____ Ear lobe

_____ Bridge of the nose

_____ Tip of the nose

_____ Finger

_____ Toe

5. _____ When using the pulse oximeter, the probe should be placed over a pulsating vascular bed. (True/False)

- Click **Patient Care** and then **Nurse-Client Interactions**.
- Select and view the video titled **0730: Intervention—Airway**. (*Note:* Check the virtual clock to see whether enough time has elapsed. You can use the fast-forward feature to advance the time by 2-minute intervals if the video is not yet available. Then click again on **Patient Care** and **Nurse-Client Interactions** to refresh the screen.)

6. Jacquline Catanazaro is experiencing an acute asthma attack. What has been planned to manage the onset of this attack?

7. What will the arterial blood gases determine?

- Click **Physical Assessment** and complete a head-to-toe assessment.

8. What respiratory system findings in Jacquline Catanazaro's assessment are consistent with an exacerbation of asthma?

9. Jacquline Catanazaro's lung assessment reveals the presence of wheezes. Which description is consistent with wheezes?
   a. Heard most frequently with inspiration
   b. Caused by air movement through narrowed bronchioles
   c. Caused by fluid, mucus, or pus in the small airways and alveoli
   d. Dry, creaking, grating, low-pitched sounds heard during inspiration and expiration

10. Jacquline Catanazaro's lung assessment reveals the presence of crackles. Which description is consistent with crackles?
    a. Bubbling sounds that are similar to the sound produced when strands of hair are rubbed between the fingers
    b. Caused by inflammation of the respiratory tree
    c. Loud machine-like sounds heard over the anterior chest wall
    d. High-pitched musical sounds heard with inspiration or expiration

11. Are there any other significant system findings?

- Click **Chart** and then **402** to view Jacquline Catanazaro's chart.
- Click the **Physician's Orders** tab and note the admission orders for Monday at 1600.
- Click **Return to Room 402** and then click the **Drug** icon at the bottom of the screen.
- Review the information for the drugs that have been prescribed for Jacquline Catanazaro.

12. What are the doses and routes of administration for each of the medications ordered to manage Jacquline Catanazaro's respiratory condition?

    a. Beclomethasone:

    b. Albuterol:

    c. Ipratropium bromide:

13. Below, match each prescribed medication with its correct mode of action.

Medication	Mode of Action
_____ Beclomethasone	a. Relief of bronchospasms
_____ Albuterol	b. Reduction of bronchial inflammation
_____ Ipratropium bromide	c. Control of secretions

14. When reinforcing patient instructions concerning the use of beclomethasone, which should be emphasized in the list of potential side effects associated with the medication? Select all that apply.

_____ Throat irritation

_____ Cough

_____ Nausea

_____ Nasal dryness

_____ Skin rash

- Click **Return to Room 402**.
- Click **Chart** and then **402**.
- Click the **Physician's Orders** tab and review the orders for Monday at 1600.

15. What tests and/or assessments will be used to monitor Jacquline Catanazaro's respiratory status?

16. What medication has been ordered for Jacquline Catanazaro?

17. What are the classification and mode of action for this medication?

18. List several clinical manifestations that would indicate improvement in Jacquline Catanazaro's condition.

Implementing a Plan of Care for the Asthmatic Patient with Psychological Complications

Reading Assignment: Care of the Patient with a Respiratory Disorder (Chapter 50)

Patient: Jacquline Catanazaro, Room 402

Objectives:

1. Evaluate the impact of the patient's social history on anticipated compliance after discharge.
2. Identify the elements to be incorporated into the teaching plan in preparation for discharge.
3. Identify priorities in nursing diagnoses for the patient experiencing coexisting psychological and physiologic conditions.

Exercise 1

Writing Activity

15 minutes

1. _____ is a severe asthmatic attack that fails to respond to the normal treatment plan.

2. What extrinsic factors are associated with an asthmatic attack? Select all that apply.

   _____ Infection

   _____ Dust

   _____ Pollen

   _____ Exercise

   _____ Foods

3. When caring for the patient with asthma, it is imperative for the nurse to recognize that which manifestations are associated with hypoxia? Select all that apply.

   _____ Restlessness

   _____ Tachycardia

   _____ Fever

   _____ Bradycardia

   _____ Confusion

4. What is the prognosis for asthma?

5. Match the columns below to show which characteristics are related to each condition.
   (*Note:* Conditions may be used more than one time.)

Characteristic	Condition
_____ Airflow on exhalation is slowed or stopped by overinflated alveoli.	a. Chronic bronchitis
_____ Excessive amount of mucus obstructs airways.	b. Asthma
_____ Exposure to irritants causes the bronchial smooth muscles to constrict.	c. Emphysema
_____ Disease process results in impaired ciliary function.	

6. Theophylline has which effect in the body?
   a. Mucolytic
   b. Reducing inflammation
   c. Bronchdilating
   d. Antibacterial

7. Match each drug with its correct classification.

Drug	Classification
_____ Salmeterol	a. Corticosteroid
_____ Fluticasone	b. Long-acting beta receptor agonist
_____ Adrenalin	c. Short-acting beta receptor agonist
_____ Albuterol	d. Bronchodilator

Exercise 2

Virtual Hospital Activity

45 minutes

- Sign in to work at Pacific View Regional Hospital for Period of Care 2. (*Note:* If you are already in the Virtual Hospital from a previous exercise, click **Leave the Floor** and then **Restart the Program** to get to the sign-in window.)
- From the Patient List, select Jacquline Catanazaro (Room 402).
- Click **Get Report** and read the Clinical Report.

1. Describe the psychological behaviors documented in the two change-of-shift reports.

2. How do these psychological behaviors affect Jacquline Catanazaro's condition?

- Click **Go to Nurses' Station** and then **402**.
- Read the **Initial Observations**.
- Click **Take Vital Signs** and review the findings.
- Click **Patient Care** and complete a head-to-toe assessment.
- Next, click **Nurse-Client Interactions**.
- Select and view the video titled **1115: Assessment—Readiness to Learn**. (*Note:* Check the virtual clock to see whether enough time has elapsed. You can use the fast-forward feature to advance the time by 2-minute intervals if the video is not yet available. Then click again on **Patient Care** and **Nurse-Client Interactions** to refresh the screen.)

3. What is the focus of the video interaction?

4. Do social supports appear to be available for Jacquline Catanazaro?

5. What are the priorities of care associated with Jacquline Catanazaro's psychosocial needs?

6. What are the priorities of care associated with Jacquline Catanazaro's physiologic needs?

- Click **Chart** and then **402** to view Jacquline Catanazaro's chart.
- Click the **History and Physical** tab and review the information given.

7. List some significant issues identified in Jacquline Catanazaro's medical history.

8. List several significant issues identified in Jacquline Catanazaro's social history.

9. Describe the interrelationships among the medical and social elements in Jacquline Catanazaro's history.

10. What factors in Jacquline Catanazaro's medical history will significantly affect her discharge?

11. How does Jacquline Catanazaro's mental health affect her physical health?

- Still in the patient's chart, click the **Consultations** tab and review the information given.

12. Discuss the plan identified in the Psychiatric Consult report.

- Click the **Patient Education** tab and review the education goals listed.

13. What educational goals are identified?

14. Who should be included in the teaching plan for Jacquline Catanazaro?

15. When preparing for discharge, the nurse will need to ensure that Jacquline Catanazaro understands the medications that have been prescribed. What information should be included concerning the prescribed corticosteroids?
    a. Take with food to minimize stomach upset.
    b. Avoid taking with milk.
    c. Do not use OTC cold preparations.
    d. Take medications immediately upon awakening each morning.

16. When reviewing potential side effects of the prescribed medications, which reactions is associated with ipratropium and should be reported to the physician?
    a. Acute eye pain
    b. Dry mouth
    c. Cough
    d. Nasal irritation

17. Which two nursing diagnoses are priorities for the patient at this point in her care?

LESSON

27

Care and Treatment of the Patient with Complications of Cancer

Reading Assignment: Care of the Patient with Cancer (Chapter 58)

Patient: Pablo Rodriguez, Room 405

Objectives:

1. Discuss complications associated with cancer.
2. Discuss the management of the patient experiencing dehydration secondary to chemotherapy.
3. Prioritize the problems of the patient experiencing complications of cancer.
4. Evaluate abnormal laboratory findings.

Exercise 1

Virtual Hospital Activity

15 minutes

- Sign in to work at Pacific View Regional Hospital for Period of Care 2. (*Note:* If you are already in the virtual hospital from a previous exercise, click **Leave the Floor** and then **Restart the Program** to get to the sign-in window.)
- From the Patient List, select Pablo Rodriguez (Room 405).
- Click **Get Report** and read the Clinical Report.
- Click **Go to Nurses' Station**.
- Click **Chart** and then **405** to view Pablo Rodriguez's chart.
- Click the **Emergency Department** tab and review the information given.

1. What are the four priorities identified in the change-of-shift report?

2. Why was Pablo Rodriguez admitted to the hospital?

3. What has caused this condition?

4. What findings support this diagnosis?

5. How was his condition initially managed in the emergency department?

6. What types of interventions (nursing and medical) may be implemented to manage his care?

7. What should be monitored to determine the degree of dehydration?

8. What are the primary goals for this hospitalization?

- Click the **History and Physical** tab and read the report.

9. List the impressions identified in the History and Physical.

Exercise 2

Virtual Hospital Activity

30 minutes

- Sign in to work at Pacific View Regional Hospital for Period of Care 2. (*Note:* If you are already in the virtual hospital from a previous exercise, click **Leave the Floor** and then **Restart the Program** to get to the sign-in window.)
- From the Patient List, select Pablo Rodriguez (Room 405).
- Click **Go to Nurses' Station**.
- Click **405** at the bottom of the screen to enter Pablo Rodriguez's room.
- Click **Take Vital Signs** and then **Clinical Alerts** and review the information given.
- Read the **Initial Observations** and read the notes.
- Click **Patient Care** and complete a head-to-toe assessment.

1. What current assessment findings support the diagnosis of dehydration?

- Click **Chart** and then **405** to view Pablo Rodriguez's chart.
- Click the **Physician's Orders** tab and review the orders since Tuesday at 2300.

2. Which medications have been ordered to manage Pablo Rodriguez's nausea?

- Click **Return to Room 405** and then click the **Drug** icon at the bottom of the screen.
- Review the medications you identified in the previous question.

3. To which drug classification does ondansetron hydrochloride belong?

4. What side effects of ondansetron could be problematic, considering Pablo Rodriguez's health concerns?

5. What is metoclopramide's mechanism of action?

- Click **Return to Room 405**.
- Once again, click **Chart** and then **405**.
- This time, click the **Laboratory Reports** tab and review the report given.

6. Review and discuss any significant findings in the CBC results.

7. Consider the clinical presentation of Pablo Rodriguez. Which manifestations may be attributed to his complete blood cell test results? Select all that apply.

_____ Nausea

_____ Vomiting

_____ Weaknesses

_____ Fatigue

_____ Reduced skin turgor

8. Are there any significant findings in the electrolyte profile?

9. Identify two of the nursing diagnoses that have the highest priority related to Pablo Rodriguez's admitting diagnosis.

Exercise 3

Virtual Hospital Activity

30 minutes

- Sign in to work at Pacific View Regional Hospital for Period of Care 2. (*Note:* If you are already in the virtual hospital from a previous exercise, click **Leave the Floor** and then **Restart the Program** to get to the sign-in window.)
- From the Patient List, select Pablo Rodriguez (Room 405).
- Click **Get Report** and read the Clinical Report.
- Click **Go to Nurses' Station** and then **405** at the bottom of the screen to enter Pablo Rodriguez's room.
- Click **Take Vital Signs** and review the information given.

1. How does Pablo Rodriguez rate his pain?

- Click **MAR** and then tab **405** to review the medications ordered for Pablo Rodriguez.

2. What medications have been ordered to manage Pablo Rodriguez's pain?

3. What is the advantage of this type of dosing?

4. List some opioids that may be prescribed to manage the pain associated with advanced cancer.

5. When administering opioids to manage Pablo Rodriguez's pain, the nurse must understand that which manifestations are common side effects associated with their use? Select all that apply.

_____ Diarrhea

_____ Constipation

_____ Bradycardia

_____ Rash

_____ Respiratory depression

_____ Hyperthermia

_____ Vomiting

6. List several nonopioid medications that can be administered to reduce mild to moderate pain associated with cancer.

7. Discuss medication scheduling techniques that effectively manage pain.

8. As previously stated, Pablo Rodriguez has been experiencing anxiety. Discuss the relationship between pain and anxiety.

9. In addition to medication therapy, what other interventions may be used to manage pain?

10. What factors may influence a patient's perception of and/or reaction to pain?

- Click **Return to Room 405**.
- Click **Patient Care** and then **Nurse-Client Interactions**.
- Select and view the video titled **1130: Family Interaction**. (*Note:* Check ʒ virtual clock to see whether enough time has elapsed. You can use the fast-forward feature to advⁿ ⁻e the time by 2-minute intervals if the video is not yet available. Then click again on **Patient Car** ₋ıd **Nurse-Client Interactions** to refresh the screen.)

11. What is the underlying message Pablo Rodriguez is attempting to communicate to his daughter?
    a. He is too tired to attend her wedding.
    b. The enema has made him feel better.
    c. He is ready to give in to the disease and die.
    d. The enema has caused him pain.

12. Does the response by Pablo Rodriguez's daughter indicate a readiness to accept her f₋ʰer's condition?

13. _____ Pablo Rodriguez will be allowed to make the decision to forgo further treatment without the approval of his immediate family. (True/False)

14. Identify referrals that may be beneficial for Pablo Rodriguez and his family at this time.

Care and Treatment of the Patient with Cancer

Reading Assignment: Care of the Patient with Cancer (Chapter 58)

Patient: Pablo Rodriguez, Room 405

Objectives:

1. Identify the physiologic changes associated with the diagnosis of cancer.
2. List risk factors for the development of cancer.
3. Identify the tests that may be used to diagnose cancer.
4. Define metastasis.

Exercise 1

Writing Activity

30 minutes

1. Which foods have been shown to reduce the risk for cancer? Select all that apply.

   _____ Broccoli

   _____ Lettuce

   _____ Bananas

   _____ Carrots

   _____ Grapefruit

   _____ Tomatoes

2. Consuming at least _____ servings of fruits and vegetables per day has been shown to reduce the risk for cancer.

3. Smokeless tobacco increases the risk of developing cancer of the _____,

   _____, _____, and _____.

4. A variety of diagnostic tests may be utilized to assess for potential malignancies. Match each diagnostic test with its correct description.

Diagnostic Test	**Description**
_____ Computed tomography	a. Noninvasive, high-frequency sound waves are used to examine external body structures.
_____ Radioisotope studies	b. A computer is used to process radiofrequency energy waves to assess spinal lesions, as well as cardiovascular and soft tissue abnormalities.
_____ Ultrasound testing	
_____ Magnetic resonance imaging	c. Radiographs and computed scanning are used to provide images of structures at differing angles.
	d. A substance is injected or ingested; then the uptake is evaluated to identify areas of concern.

5. Which characteristics are associated with a benign growth? Select all that apply.

_____ Grows rapidly

_____ Smooth and well-defined

_____ Immobile when palpated

_____ Often recurs after removal

_____ Crowds normal tissue

_____ Remains localized

6. Match each diagnostic laboratory test with the type of cancer it is used to detect.

Diagnostic Test	Type of Cancer Detected
_____ Serum calcitonin levels	a. Thyroid, breast, and oat (small) cell cancer in the lung
_____ Carcinoembryonic antigen	b. Gynecologic and pancreatic cancers
_____ PSA	c. Prostate cancer
_____ CA-125	d. Colorectal cancer

7. The complete blood cell profile of a patient diagnosed with cancer shows a reduction in the number of circulating platelets. Which term is used to describe this condition?
   a. Leukopenia
   b. Thrombocytopenia
   c. Anemia
   d. Neutropenia

8. Discuss the use of radiation treatments to manage cancer.

9. What is the mode of action for chemotherapy drugs?

10. Sometimes cancer is described as *metastatic*. What does this mean?

11. How does metastasis occur?

12. Use of the immune system to counteract the destruction of cancer cells is known as

   _____. _____ may be used to remove a tumor, lesion, and surrounding malignant tissue.

13. Indicate whether each statement is true or false.

   a. _____ Alopecia in patients undergoing chemotherapy results from damage to the hair follicle.

   b. _____ Alopecia is permanent.

   c. _____ Hair that regrows may be of a different color and/or texture than original hair.

14. List and discuss the complications involving the gastrointestinal system associated with the administration of chemotherapy.

15. Why is the patient with cancer at risk for developing nutritional problems?

16. For what nutritional disturbances is the patient with cancer at risk?

Exercise 2

Virtual Hospital Activity

30 minutes

- Sign in to work at Pacific View Regional Hospital for Period of Care 4. (*Note:* If you are already in the virtual hospital from a previous exercise, click **Leave the Floor** and then **Restart the Program** to get to the sign-in window.)
- Click **Chart** and then **405** to view Pablo Rodriguez's chart. (*Remember:* You are not able to visit patients or administer medications during Period of Care 4. You are only able to review patient records.)
- Click the **Nursing Admission** tab and review the information given.

1. What is Pablo Rodriguez's medical diagnosis?

2. According to the Nursing Admission, how does the patient describe his prognosis?

3. When was Pablo Rodriguez diagnosed with lung cancer?

- Click the **History and Physical** tab and review the reports.

4. How has Pablo Rodriguez's cancer been treated?

5. Does he have any family history of cancer?

6. Does his social history contain any risk factors for his diagnosis of lung cancer?

7. What psychosocial changes have resulted in his life because of the cancer?

8. Discuss the physical changes that have taken place as a result of Pablo Rodriguez's cancer.

9. Discuss Pablo Rodriguez's emotional readiness for death.

10. What emotional concerns have been voiced by the patient?

11. What therapeutic behaviors by the nurse are essential at this time?

12. What factors may put Pablo Rodriguez at risk for infection?

13. In addition to the nausea and vomiting, is Pablo Rodriguez suffering from any other complications of the gastrointestinal system?

14. Has Pablo Rodriguez experienced any nutritional disturbances during his illness?

LESSON **29**

Assessment of the Patient with Gastrointestinal Complications

Reading Assignment: Care of the Patient with a Gastrointestinal Disorder (Chapter 46)

Patient: Piya Jordan, Room 403

Objectives:

1. Identify clinical manifestations and causes of intestinal obstructions.
2. Identify priorities in nursing diagnoses for the patient experiencing an intestinal obstruction.
3. Explain operative measures used in cases of intestinal obstruction.
4. Identify common gastrointestinal disorders.
5. Identify tests used in the diagnosis of gastrointestinal disorders.
6. List medications used in the management of gastrointestinal disorders.

Exercise 1

Writing Activity

15 minutes

1. Describe the two types of intestinal obstructions.

   a. Mechanical obstruction:

   b. Nonmechanical obstruction:

2. The signs and symptoms associated with a bowel obstruction will be determined by the

   _____ and _____ of _____.

3. When caring for a patient suspected of having an intestinal obstruction, which manifestations would be considered early symptoms? Select all that apply.

   _____   Loud bowel sounds

   _____   High-pitched bowel sounds

   _____   Vomiting

   _____   Constipation

   _____   Absence of bowel sounds

   _____   Frequent bowel sounds

   _____   Abdominal pain

4. Identify several causes of mechanical intestinal obstructions.

5. Which are causes associated with nonmechanical intestinal obstructions? Select all that apply.

_____   Complications from surgery

_____   Bowel tumors

_____   Electrolyte abnormalities

_____   Thoracic spinal trauma

_____   Lumbar spinal trauma

_____   Embolism or atherosclerosis of the mesenteric arteries

_____   Impacted feces

6. _____   Paralytic ileus is the most common type of nonmechanical intestinal obstruction. (True/False)

7. Which symptoms, if present, can be associated with a paralytic ileus? Select all that apply.

_____   Increased abdominal girth

_____   Distention

_____   Urinary frequency

_____   Elevated white blood cell count

_____   Vomiting

8. Which interventions are done to reduce the risk for developing a paralytic ileus? Select all that apply.

_____   Abdominal assessment

_____   IV therapy

_____   Maintenance of NG tube

_____   Increase in patient activity

_____   Deep breathing exercises

Exercise 2

Writing Activity

30 minutes

1. Match each diagnostic test with its correct description.

Diagnostic Test	**Description**
_____ Upper gastrointestinal study	a. Aspiration and review of stomach contents to determine acid production
_____ Tube gastric analysis	
_____ Esophagogastroduodenoscopy	b. Radiographs of the lower esophagus, stomach, and duodenum using barium sulfate as a contrast medium
_____ Lower GI endoscopy	c. Visualization of the upper GI tract by a flexible scope
_____ Bernstein test	d. An acid-perfusion test using hydrochloric acid
	e. Assessment of the lower GI tract with a scope

2. What is a KUB?

3. When reinforcing education to a patient diagnosed with gastroesophageal reflux disease (GERD), what information should be emphasized in the teaching session? Select all that apply.

_____ Eat a low-fat, low-protein diet

_____ Avoid eating 4 to 6 hours before bedtime

_____ Remain upright for 1 to 2 hours after meals

_____ Avoid eating in bed

_____ Eat 4 to 6 small meals per day

_____ Reduce caffeine intake

4. Match each gastrointestinal disorder with its correct description.

Gastrointestinal Disorder

_____ GERD

_____ Candidiasis

_____ Gastritis

_____ Irritable bowel syndrome

_____ Ulcerative colitis

_____ Crohn's disease

_____ Diverticulosis

Description

a. The presence of pouchlike herniations through the muscular layers of the colon

b. Characterized by inflammation of segments of the GI tract, resulting in a cobblestone-like appearance of the mucosa

c. Episodic bowel dysfunction characterized by intestinal pain, disturbed defecation, or abdominal distention

d. The formation of tiny abscesses on mucosa and submucosa of the colon, producing drainage and sloughing of the mucosa and subsequent ulcerations

e. The backward flow of stomach acid into the esophagus

f. A fungal infection presenting as white patches on the mucous membranes

g. Inflammation of the lining of the stomach

5. Match each gastrointestinal medication with its correct classification.

Medication

_____ Maalox

_____ Famotidine

_____ Omeprazole

_____ Sucrafate

_____ Misoprostol

Classification

a. Proton pump inhibitor

b. Antacid

c. Prostaglandin

d. Mucosal protectant agent

e. Histamine H_2 receptor blocker

6. Which alternative therapies should be avoided because they can cause GI upset? Select all that apply.

_____ Comfrey

_____ Digitalis leaf

_____ Ginger

_____ Golden seal

_____ Spearmint extract

7. Gastrointestinal disorders may be more prevalent in certain ethnic groups. Which ethnic group has a higher incidence of inflammatory bowel disease?
   a. Ashkenazi Jewish
   b. African-American
   c. Asian-American
   d. Americans of Middle Eastern descent

8. A common cause of peptic ulcer disease is the presence of which microorganism?

9. What is a colectomy? What is a colostomy?

Exercise 3

Virtual Hospital Activity

15 minutes

- Sign in to work at Pacific View Regional Hospital for Period of Care 1. (*Note:* If you are already in the virtual hospital from a previous exercise, click **Leave the Floor** and then **Restart the Program** to get to the sign-in window.)
- From the Patient List, select Piya Jordan (Room 403).
- Click **Get Report** and read the Clinical Report.
- Click **Go to Nurse's Station**.
- Click **Chart** and then **403** to view Piya Jordan's chart.
- Click the **Emergency Department** tab and review the information given.

1. What are Piya Jordan's primary complaints upon arrival to the emergency department?

2. What are Piya Jordan's vital signs at admission?

HR:

T:

RR:

BP:

3. What can Piya Jordan's hypotension most likely be attributed to?
   a. The presence of infection
   b. An elevation in blood glucose values
   c. Hypokalemia
   d. Dehydration

4. What diagnostic tests were ordered for Piya Jordan in the emergency department?

5. According to the ED physician's progress notes, what are the abnormal findings on the physical assessment that support a potential bowel obstruction?

6. What are the treatment goals of the care for a patient experiencing an intestinal obstruction?

7. Initial management of the patient's condition included the placement of a nasogastric (NG) tube. The NG tube can serve a variety of functions. Match each function with its correct description.

Function	Description
_____ Decompression	a. Irrigation of the stomach, used in cases of active bleeding, poisoning, or gastric dilation
_____ Feeding	
	b. Removal of secretions and gases from the GI tract
_____ Compression	
	c. Internal application of pressure by means of an inflated balloon to prevent internal GI hemorrhage
_____ Lavage	
	d. Instillation of liquid supplements into the stomach

8. Piya Jordan has had the NG tube inserted for _____.

• Click **Surgical Reports** in the chart.

9. Piya Jordan has had a right hemicolectomy. Which description of the procedure is most accurate?
   a. Resection of ascending colon and hepatic flexure; ileum anastomosed to transverse colon
   b. Resection of the splenic flexure, descending colon, and sigmoid colon; transverse colon anastomosed to rectum
   c. Resection of part of the descending colon, the sigmoid colon, and upper rectum; descending colon anastomosed to remaining rectum
   d. Resection of the descending colon, the sigmoid colon, and upper rectum to the ileum and anastomosed to the transverse colon

• Click **Return to Nurses' Station**.
• Click **Chart** and go to Piya Jordan's chart.
• Review the **Physician's Orders** for Wednesday at 0730.

10. According to the Initial Observations, blood is being administered to Piya Jordan. What laboratory results will necessitate close observation to determine the effectiveness of this intervention?

11. What will the nurse need to monitor concerning the blood transfusion?

12. Piya Jordan has remained NPO since the surgery. What information will the nurse need to monitor to ensure she is adequately hydrated?

13. Which position will be most therapeutic to Piya Jordan in the postoperative period?
    a. Semi-Fowler's
    b. Fowler's
    c. Prone
    d. Side-lying

LESSON 30

Colorectal Cancer and Care of the Patient After Gastrointestinal Surgery

Reading Assignment: Care of the Surgical Patient (Chapter 43)
Care of the Patient with a Gastrointestinal Disorder (Chapter 46)

Patient: Piya Jordan, Room 403

Objectives:

1. Identify risk factors associated with the development of colorectal cancer.
2. List the warning signs and symptoms associated with a diagnosis of colorectal cancer.
3. Identify the assessment priorities for the postoperative patient.
4. Discuss the safe use of narcotics administered in the postoperative period.
5. Discuss the potential for postoperative complications.

Exercise 1

Writing Activity

15 minutes

1. Indicate whether each statement is true or false.

    a. _____ Cancer of the colon and rectum is the second leading cause of cancer in the United States.

    b. _____ In the early stages, colorectal cancer is often asymptomatic.

2. What factors may be associated with colorectal cancer? Select all that apply.

    _____ Ulcerative colitis

    _____ Peritonitis

    _____ Diverticulosis

    _____ Elevated bacterial counts in the colon

    _____ Vegan diets

    _____ High dietary fat intake

    _____ Dietary intake high in cruciferous vegetables

3. The nurse is caring for a patient who is 36 years old. She has a family history of colon cancer. What recommendations should be provided to this patient concerning screening?
   a. Begin colonoscopy screening after age 50.
   b. Have a baseline colonoscopy before age 50.
   c. Have an initial colonoscopy before age 40 and then every 5 years after.
   d. No special screening recommendations are needed.

4. Which symptoms are associated with the later stages of colorectal cancer? Select all that apply.

    _____ Constipation

    _____ Diarrhea

    _____ Abdominal pain

    _____ Anemia

    _____ Weakness

    _____ Emaciation

5. The incidence of colorectal cancer increases in persons over age _____.

6. The 5-year survival rate for early localized colorectal cancer is _____%; for cancer that has

   spread to adjacent organs and lymph nodes, it is _____%.

7. _____ refers to weakness and emaciation associated with general ill
   health and malnutrition.

8. What details should be included in the assessment of a surgical incision?

Exercise 2

Virtual Hospital Activity

30 minutes

- Sign in to work at Pacific View Regional Hospital for Period of Care 1. (*Note:* If you are already in the
  virtual hospital from a previous exercise, click **Leave the Floor** and then **Restart the Program** to get to
  the sign-in window.)
- From the Patient List, select Piya Jordan (Room 403).
- Click **Get Report** and read the Clinical Report.
- Click **Go to Nurses' Station** and then click the **Drug** icon. Find the entry for meperidine and review.

1. Based on your review of the shift report, which care factors appear to be of high priority?

2. The assessment findings of which of the patient's body systems demonstrate the potential for
   developing postoperative complications?
   a. Respiratory system
   b. Renal system
   c. Integumentary system
   d. Reproductive system

- Click **Return to Nurses' Station**.
- Click **403** and read the **Initial Observations**.
- Click **Take Vital Signs** and then on **Clinical Alerts** and review the information given.
- Click **Patient Care** and complete a head-to-toe assessment.

3. Discuss the proper assessment of bowel sounds for this patient.

4. What is the purpose of the Jackson-Pratt drain? How long will it need to be in place for Piya Jordan?

5. When the nurse is providing care for Piya Jordan, what should be monitored and recorded regarding the NG tube?

6. Piya Jordan has a reduced aeration to the left lower lobe. What interventions can promote improved aeration and a reduction in potential complications?

- Click **Chart** and then **403** to view Piya Jordan's chart.
- Click the **Nurse's Notes** tab and review the information given.

7. According to the Wednesday 0630 Nurse's Notes, Piya Jordan's meperidine PCA was discontinued because of suspicions of toxicity. Which clinical manifestations are associated with meperidine toxicity? Select all that apply.

_____ Respiratory depression

_____ Systolic hypertension

_____ Clammy skin

_____ Cyanosis

_____ Stupor

_____ Coma

_____ Diarrhea

8. In the event that pharmacologic intervention is needed to treat meperidine overdosage, which medication may be administered?
   a. Prochorperazine
   b. Promethazine
   c. Famotidine
   d. Naloxone

9. The nurse should observe for which possible side effects and adverse effects associated with meperidine? Select all that apply.

_____ Nausea/vomiting

_____ Diarrhea

_____ Bradycardia

_____ Flushed face

_____ Euphoria

- Click **Return to Room 403**.
- Click **Physical Assessment** and complete a head-to-toe assessment.

10. The clinical report at 0730 indicates Piya Jordan is experiencing which possible adverse effects from meperidine? Select all that apply.

_____   Confusion

_____   Serosanguinous drainage from the Jackson-Pratt drain

_____   Restlessness

_____   Agitation

_____   Brown drainage from the nasogastric tube

- Click **Patient Care** and then **Nurse-Client Interactions**.
- Select and view the video titled **0735: Pain—Adverse Drug Event**. (*Note:* Check the virtual clock to see whether enough time has elapsed. You can use the fast-forward feature to advance the time by 2-minute intervals if the video is not yet available. Then click again on **Patient Care** and **Nurse-Client Interactions** to refresh the screen.)

11. What problems were encountered during the previous evening with regard to the use of the PCA pump?

12. What patient/family concerns during the video indicate the need for education?

13. What issues does the nurse need to address with Piya Jordan's daughter in particular?

Exercise 3

Virtual Hospital Activity

15 minutes

- Sign in to work at Pacific View Regional Hospital for Period of Care 3. (*Note:* If you are already in the virtual hospital from a previous exercise, click **Leave the Floor** and then **Restart the Program** to get to the sign-in window.)
- From the Patient List, select Piya Jordan (Room 403).
- Click **Get Report** and read the Clinical Report.
- Click **Go to Nurses' Station**.
- Click **403** at the bottom of the screen to enter the patient's room.
- Read the **Initial Observations**.

1. Have there been any changes in mental status since Period of Care 1?

2. What changes have been made to the type and/or administration of Piya Jordan's pain medication?

3. How does Piya Jordan rate her pain at this time?

- Click **Chart** and then **403** to view Piya Jordan's chart.
- Click the **Surgical Reports** tab and review the reports.

4. What type of surgery was planned for Piya Jordan? What surgical procedure was actually completed?

5. What are the most common complications associated with the surgery performed on Piya Jordan? Select all that apply.

_____   Hemorrhage

_____   Infection

_____   Blood loss

_____   Pneumonia

_____   Wound dehiscence

_____   Blood clots

_____   Paralytic ileus

6. What is Piya Jordan's postoperative diagnosis?